CU00545994

THE PORTABLE GREG EVERETT

COLLECTED
ARTICLES
2005-2012

Copyright 2005-2012 Greg Everett

Published by Catalyst Athletics, Inc. All rights reserved.
No part of this book may be reproduced in any form
without prior written consent from the publisher.

ISBN-13: 978-0-9800111-3-5
ISBN-10: 0-9800111-3-2

APOD

Catalyst Athletics, Inc.
www.catalystathletics.com

THE PORTABLE GREG EVERETT

COLLECTED ARTICLES 2005-2012

CONTENTS

INTRODUCTION

This book was largely created on a whim; I never planned to put out such a collection, but having received quite a few requests for it, I decided it made sense. What I've done is simply pulled together some of the better articles I've written for Catalyst Athletics over the last seven years. Some originally appeared in the Performance Menu journal, and others appeared on the Catalyst Athletics website article section or blog.

It was an interesting process reading some of these articles again for the first time in years—I forgot that several of them existed. At the time of this writing, the Performance Menu is in its 8th year and 86th issue—that's almost 400 articles. There are over 150 more articles on the Catalyst Athletics website. With all of that content going through my head at some point, whether when being written or edited, my memory of it is not particularly sharp, so often I felt like I was reading an article for the first time myself.

I've also included content from the Ask Greg column of the Performance Menu. Please forgive the spelling, grammar and formatting of the readers' emails.

I hope you find this collection interesting, enlightening, entertaining or in some fashion enjoyable. It's been a lot of work over the years producing this content, but I'm grateful every day to have an appreciative audience to produce it for.

—Greg Everett
March 16 2012

SIX TRUTHS OF WEIGHTLIFTING TECHNIQUE

When it comes to weightlifting technique, there are disagreements. Some are legitimate, some are questionable, and a few are downright silly. But when you sift through it all, there are a few universal Truths when it comes to the snatch and clean. If you can make these following six things happen with a given technical style, you can probably make it work for you.

Truth 1: The lifter and barbell system must remain balanced over the feet. This is pretty simple. If the balance of the system doesn't remain over the feet, the combined weight of the bar and lifter will not be supported by the base and it will fall over. This is basically an average measure—the actual balance over the foot isn't exactly the same throughout a given lift, but it must end up being essentially balanced on average. If it diverges too much at any given point, it will be more than the lifter can compensate for, and the result will be the entire system being pulled forward or backward out of balance. There is actually a bit of latitude here. It's possible to perform a snatch or clean with a backward or even forward jump as long as you can re-establish the balance over the newly positioned base. However, there is a limit to how much this can be done, and any degree of horizontal movement, in particular in a forward direction, makes the stabilization of the bar more difficult.

Truth 2: The barbell and lifter must remain in close proximity to each other.
This seems pretty obvious like Truth One, but this Truth is violated so commonly that it warrants emphasis. I like to illustrate this point by asking people what they would do if I asked them to pick up a barbell and then rolled it away from them. Everyone either answers that they would walk up to the bar or roll the bar back to themselves—in this extreme example, no one fails to recognize that the closer the bar is, the easier it is to lift. When we're talking about a more complex movement like the snatch or clean, the effect of distance between the bar and body is magnified; that is, extremely small distances can create big problems. I prefer to have the barbell as close to the lifter as possible without making contact until the appropriate point of contact during the final explosion effort (hips for the snatch, high upper thigh for the clean), but would rather have it in light contact earlier

than be considerably distant.

Truth 3: There must be no time wasted at the top of the pull.

You can argue about either the elevation of the bar or the pull under the bar being more important than the other, but you can't deny that any time spent in an extended position following the point of producing maximal acceleration is limiting the lifter's ability to relocate under the bar. That is, whether you want to focus on lifting the bar or getting under it (or, a novel idea, both...), you have to transition between accelerating the bar upward and accelerating the body downward as quickly as possible.

Truth 4: The relocation under the bar is an active movement

The pull or push under the bar must be as aggressive as the attempt to accelerate it upward. In effective lifting, there is no falling, dropping or catching. There is pulling, pushing, squatting and splitting—the relocation of the lifter under the bar is just as active as the rest of the lift, and a lack of aggression in this phase of the lift will ensure a lifter fails to maximize his or her potential.

Truth 5: The receiving position must be stable and strong.

You can argue with regard to the snatch or jerk about how many degrees of internal or external rotation of the humerus is correct, what the shoulder blades should be doing, and how the hands should be holding the bar, but all that matters is that you establish the position that best allows you to support the weight and stand up with it. This position will vary somewhat among lifters based on anatomical peculiarities, flexibility, etc. The rack position of the clean similarly will look different among lifters, but in any case, the bar must be supported securely on the trunk, not in the hands and arms, and the position must allow optimal posture in the squat position.

Truth 6: Consistency is more important than the actual technical style.

No two athletes lift exactly the same way. Some use the same basic style, but every lifter has his or her own technical idiosyncrasies for better or worse. In the long term, it's more important that a lifter perform the lifts as consistently as possible relative to him- or herself than it is to perform the lifts with a certain technical style (assuming the style is within the range of acceptable). If a lifter is much better with an emphasis on hip extension, his snatch or clean will look different than a lifter who is better at producing a powerful downward punch of the legs along with the hip explosion. If those styles are truly what works best for each lifter, each lifter is maximizing his ability and attempts to mimic another technical style will limit that ability to lift as much as possible. Each lifter should strive to optimize the technique that proves to be most effective, and then make that optimized technique second nature through high volumes of practice and training over time.

THE PORTABLE GREG EVERETT

HIPS, MEET BAR

Some topics seem to generate more heat that others, and for some reason, the question of how a barbell should come into contact with the body during the snatch and clean seems to get some people extraordinarily wound up. I personally don't lose any sleep over how anyone else lifts or teaches the lifts. I may agree or disagree, but I don't let it upset me too much. The following will undoubtedly further upset the same people who are already upset.

In my humble opinion, there is more than one way to be successful with regard to weightlifting technique. I mean this more in the sense that different technical styles are better suited to different lifters; for a given lifter, one approach will be most effective, and lifters will naturally gravitate toward that style. This is how you end up with technique like Vardanian, Dimas, Sagir, Popov, et al. They weren't taught to lift with the peculiarities that characterize their lifting technique; rather, they naturally performed the lifts in such a manner and found it successful, or they intuitively adjusted over time their approach to find the most effective style. Others trying to mimic it are rarely if ever successful.

When it comes to the barbell's contact with the body during the extension of the snatch and clean, it seems the issue has been divided into two camps, which in my opinion are not accurately representative of what's happening, but exist nonetheless: brush and bang.

Each camp has characterized the other, and I think this is where much of the disagreement comes from: neither has characterized the other accurately. The bang crowd believes the brush crowd encourages lifters to drag the bar up the body as they extend perfectly vertically with excessive ankle extension and a big shrug and hesitation at the top; the brush crowd believes the bang crowd encourages lifters to allow the bar to stay away from the body too far so the hips can be slammed into it and kick the bar forward. In cases in which either is actually being done as described, I believe it's the result of misinterpretation or misunderstanding.

There seems to be a sense as well that the bang is a new, modern technique, while the brush is some artifact of the 60s. In reality, the style of more violent hip snapping directly or nearly so into the bar has been done since at least the 80s by the Bulgarians; it's nothing new. Similarly, more of a brushing approach can be seen even among current lifters. Anyone who says "This is how all the best lifters are doing it" is wrong no matter what "this" is. Any competition at the international level showcases numerous lifting styles, and no single approach stands out as dominant, as has been the case forever. Yes, there are certain things that all successful lifters have in common, but those are so obvious and general that they don't even warrant discussion.

I have seen a number of forum posts, received numerous questions, and been told of multiple conversations about what I ostensibly teach lifters that is either unclear or incorrect. I should probably accept responsibility for this and assume that what I've written in my book, in articles or told people has simply not been clear enough. To be honest, I don't even remember how exactly I describe this part of the lift in my book after two editions and changes during multiple reprints, as my thinking on it and consequently my description has evolved somewhat since the first edition was released. That said, it hasn't changed that drastically. In any case, I will try to describe it as accurately and concisely as I can manage here. I'm sure it won't solve the misunderstanding problem entirely—getting inaccurate information off the internet is like trying to get piss out of a pool.

What I want to see with lifters ideally is pretty simple: I want the bar to remain as close to the thighs as possible without being in contact and for the shoulders to remain at least very slightly in front of the bar until the bar is up into the hips in the snatch and the upper thighs in the clean. I like to see the final explosion occur quite late in the extension and want it to be more the start of the pull under the bar than the finish of the upward elevation of the bar. This bar position is a natural result of staying over the bar until very late in the second pull—if the shoulders are in front of the bar, it's difficult to drag it up your legs, and any contact you do get inadvertently won't create much friction.

The extension of the hips must be extremely violent, and the legs should continue pushing against the platform until it's completed and no longer. This helps maintain proper balance over the feet, assists in bar elevation, and helps ensure that the force imparted to the bar is directed overwhelmingly upward rather than forward. The hips absolutely need to come into contact with the bar—in no instance should a lifter finish a pull without the bar being in full contact with the hips (or upper thighs in the clean). Any separation at this point is the result of either not completing hip extension, being too far forward on the feet and being unable to finish the pull properly as a result, or having a light weight on the bar that was swung out early in the lift.

The bar should be pushed back and up into the hips as the hips finish this snap—that is, the hips and bar should be brought together rather than the lifter reaching for the bar with the hips. This is largely a conceptual thing rather than a description of what actually happens—the hips do and must move forward toward the bar because they start behind the lifter's feet. The key is not driving them through the bar so far that vertical force is lost and the bar is pushed away, and I find that thinking of it this ways helps prevent this.

The extension should finish with the bar in contact with the hips (or upper thigh in the clean), legs approximately vertical and the hips opened beyond neutral to bring the shoulders behind the hips. While my recollection of what exactly I wrote in my book is not entirely clear, I do know that this is a point I emphasized in all printings and editions—the lift is never finished with a vertical body orientation.

This final extension of the hips is extremely quick and the hips snapping into the bar violently allows a faster reversal into the pull and squat under the bar. But this is where I think a lot of lifters get into trouble. Banging the hips into the bar in any fashion will increase your speed under the bar by allowing you to change directions faster; but if it's not done properly, it will significantly limit upward acceleration of the bar and/or push the bar forward, both of which will limit how much can be lifted.

The more of the extension the hips can perform without any contact with the bar, they faster they will be able to extend because there is less resistance. However, this has to be balanced with the need to not push the bar forward and to get adequate height on the bar. The farther forward the hips reach to the bar without contacting it, the farther the bar will get pushed out. Granted, this can be controlled to some degree with the arms during the pull under the bar, but the more horizontal force that's put onto the bar, the less vertical movement occurs.

Once the bar is in contact with the body, it should remain in contact briefly as it continues to rise. If the lifter is actively pulling the bar into the body as he or she should be to maintain proximity and balance, it will brush up the body momentarily rather than hit and immediately bounce away. To be clear, this is not the bar dragging up the body for any considerable distance or time. If the hips are extended properly, the bar will be moving up toward a body that is retreating from it (i.e. the torso is leaning back away from the bar as the bar moves up the hips).

With this kind of connection, the bar is accelerated with the hips' extension, it's able to remain traveling vertical without as much disruption, and it will actually get a bit of an upward push from the hips as they come through because they'll be moving up under the bar rather than just slamming forward against it.

Of course, this is all just my opinion, and how much that's worth is entirely up to you. As I said in the beginning, every lifter and coach needs to do what is found to be most effective for them, and if that's being done, I'm certainly not going to argue or complain about it.

IMPROVING THE CLEAN THROUGH A BETTER TURNOVER

A lot more attention tends to be paid to the third pull or turnover of the snatch than the clean, likely because the consequences of poor execution tend to be more dramatic and obvious, but the turnover of the clean deserves its own share of attention. The timing and precision of the turnover in the clean can be the difference between a make and a miss, or can prevent the recovery from being so taxing that a subsequent jerk fails.

An idea I commonly talk about with my lifters is attempting to make the clean resemble the front squat as much as possible. Even the most technically proficient and athletic lifters can front squat more than they can clean. The primary reasons are simple: it's easier to establish and maintain balance and stability, barbell positioning is ideal, and there is a longer eccentric segment.

So to make cleans more successful, we're trying to optimize balance and stability, position the barbell as well as possible in the rack, and ensure enough of an eccentric movement to create tension and a stretch reflex to aid in the recovery.

Balance and stability are affected by every part of the lift from the moment the bar leaves the platform, and arguably even before that. If the lifter's balance is off during any phase of the lift, it's very likely to remain off for the rest of the lift. If the lifter is balanced and stable early the lift, it's very likely that he or she will remain that way. With regard to the turnover specifically, the maintenance of balance requires that the lifter and barbell remain in immediate proximity to each other and extraneous movement is minimized or eliminated; this is one part of the precision element of the turnover. Consistency among lifts is also critical because it makes the movement predictable and reliable, which minimizes the need for adjustments during the very limited time during a lift.

The position of the barbell in the rack is another element of balance and stability. When taking a bar from a rack for front squats, a lifter can take his or her time establishing a perfectly secure and balanced position of the bar on the shoulders, allowing optimal posture and movement in the squat and minimal effort to maintain the bar's position. There is little or no fight to keep the bar in place during the squat and effort can be focused on actually standing up. There is also no drop of the barbell onto the lifter at any point in the squat, barring the occasional abrupt start that some lifters do that creates a small amount of separation; but even the worst offenders can't match the drop of the bar in a poorly executed clean.

Finally, the longer eccentric portion of a front squat in comparison to the clean allows for an easier recovery from the bottom due to the development of more tension and a potentially better stretch reflex. (Interestingly, one reason some lifters appear to do better with cleans than front squats is that their cleans are quick into the bottom, generating a stretch reflex, while they control the downward speed of the front squats to a greater degree, limiting the stretch reflex.)

In order to take advantage of these elements of the front squat during the clean, the turnover needs to keep the bar and body in immediate proximity to each other, bring the bar and shoulders together smoothly and precisely, and occur in as high of a squat position as possible.

Proximity of the bar and body during the turnover is maintained by moving the arms properly. This not only keeps the bar moving in the desired path, but also keeps the body close to the bar. The elbows should have been turned out from the start of the lift and kept in that orientation so that when the pull under the bar is performed, the bending elbows move out and up rather than back. The elbows moving back prematurely encourages the bar to move forward away from the body.

This movement of the arms in the initial stage of the pull under is also critical for the precision and timing of the delivery of the bar into the rack position. The actual turnover of the elbows is not a strong movement, much like in the snatch; if the body has not been accelerated downward adequately, the turning over of the elbows will not be sufficient to bring the bar and body together properly or allow the elbows to complete their spin around the bar quickly enough (or at all). This is a violent, aggressive pull against the bar to set up the turnover of the elbows, which is really just a follow-through.

This movement can be thought of as positioning the barbell near the shoulders (and the shoulders near the barbell) to establish it as an axis around which the elbows can pivot quickly. This spin of the elbows around the bar is difficult, slow and occasionally impossible if the bar and body are still in the middle of the process of moving into this position.

As a part of the movement of the elbows around the bar as the bar and shoulders come together, the shoulder blades should be retracted as the elbows come back and around, in effect rowing the bar in toward the body. This will further ensure that the bar is delivered securely into the rack position rather than winding up too far forward, or similarly problematic, forcing the lifter to lean the chest forward to reach for the bar.

Generally lifters should end up in the rack position without a full grip around the bar; that is, the bar will be resting securely on the shoulders and the hands will be at least partially open with the fingers under the bar. Lifters with adequate flexibility and convenient proportions will be able to rack the bar well with a closed grip; this is fine as long as it creates no problems such as slow completion of the turnover. In any case, the grip should be maintained until the elbows are beginning to come up from under the bar. By this point, the bar should be starting to contact the shoulders, which means it won't be able to spin freely, and the remaining turnover of the elbows will need to come with some movement of the hands on the bar (this can occur with the hand open or closed—the grip simply needs to be loosened enough to keep the elbows moving).

As a final part of the turnover, the shoulders should be pushed up into the bar to ensure the connection is made smoothly and that the bar is not allowed to simply drop onto the shoulders. Any crashing of the bar onto the body creates excessive downward force for the lifter to resist, as well as increases the likelihood of instability due to unexpected and uncontrollably sudden shifts in position. This reach of the shoulders up into the bar will also encourage the athlete to tighten up sooner and be ready to resist the weight.

Lastly, the turnover should always be completed as soon as possible; that is, the lifter should attempt to secure the bar in the rack position in as high of a squat position as possible. This is the final element of making the clean resemble the front squat: the higher the bar is racked, the sooner the lifter can establish tension in the squat, and the more of an eccentric movement can occur before the recovery. The heavier the clean, the less the lifter will be able to elevate the bar, and the lower he or she will be forced to receive it. But the principle of the effort doesn't change. Often lifters want to jump into the bottom of the squat to receive a clean despite the fact that the bar is much higher and subsequently crashes down onto the shoulders and crushes them, making the recovery far more difficult or even impossible. Commonly this problem is addressed by reducing the elevation of the bar rather than increasing the elevation of the body to meet it; that is, a lifter will start cutting his or her pull short or reducing the pull effort so the bar stops crashing. This is successful (at least in the basic sense that the lifter makes the clean) with lighter weights, but typically the lifter then fails to adjust as weights increase and simply can't elevate the bar adequately to get under it either at all or soon enough for a successful recovery from the bottom.

There are some extremely strong squatters who put up big numbers in the clean with turnovers that don't conform to the above recommendations. This can be seen as a reason to not bother with technical improvements, or it can be seen as being an unnecessary limiter of the athlete's potential. If that lifter is able to clean so much with a bar crashing down onto their shoulders in the bottom of a squat, how much more would he or she be capable of with a smooth delivery and a bit more of an eccentric component to the squat?

The specifics of how a lifter can improve the clean turnover will depend on what exactly that lifter is or isn't presently doing in the clean, but following are some exercises for technical improvements.

Rack Delivery

This is a simple drill I usually use as part of my clean teaching progression, but also use it sometimes to correct problems down the line. The lifter starts standing tall holding a barbell in the scarecrow position—bar against the chest and elbows elevated and out to the sides (the bar should hang down below the elbows rather than letting the elbows drop to lift the bar higher). From this position, the lifter will turn the bar over into the clean rack position, focusing on bringing the bar back into the body and delivering it smoothly. This can be done fairly slowly initially if necessary, but eventually should be as quick as possible without sacrificing accuracy. Generally sticking to 3-5 reps at a time is a good idea to give the shoulders a break and prevent fatigue from allowing the quality of movement to degrade. An empty bar or light technique bar will usually be as much weight as anyone can manage (note that some weight is necessary for this to work—no PVC pipes or wooden dowels).

Muscle Clean

The muscle clean is a simple way to teach and practice the upper body movement of the clean turnover. Watch that you or your athletes don't overload it; excessive weight will just encourage a return to existing bad habits. Focus should be on keeping the elbows turned out to the sides and elevating them maximally and to the sides before turning the arms over; retracting the shoulder blades and bringing the bar back in to the shoulders as the elbows move around the bar; keeping the chest up rather than reaching for the bar by leaning forward; properly timing the release of the grip to maintain connection to the bar and secure placement on the shoulders; smooth connection of the bar to the shoulders with no crashing. Work with 3-5 reps per set at a weight that allows perfect movement for all reps. This can also be done from the hang or blocks.

Tall Clean

The tall clean can be helpful to allow focus on only the pull under the bar, encourage better turnover speed, and bolster confidence. I prefer to start the tall clean on flat feet rather than on the toes because the position and balance are more similar to what they should be in the clean. The goal should be to rack the barbell as high and as smoothly as possible, and to establish tightness in the squat position immediately for a strong receipt and recovery. This can also be done with power cleans or as a tall power clean + tall clean complex.

Power Clean

There is definitely some disagreement about the use of the power clean by weightlifters, as well as disagreement about how exactly it should be performed. In short, my opinion is that the power clean should be no different than the clean other than the height at which the lifter stops squatting down after receiving the bar. The power clean can help encourage a more forceful upward extension and more aggressive turnover, as well as encouraging the lifter to meet the bar both in a high position as well as learning to immediately tighten the body to resist and support the bar.

Block / Hang Clean

Cleans from blocks or from the hang are similar to power cleans in the sense that they encourage a faster and more aggressive turnover. They will also help develop better explosiveness at the top of the pull for better bar acceleration and height in the clean.

Muscle Clean + Clean

The muscle clean can be combined with the clean (or power clean or tall clean) to help incorporate the improved turnover movement with the lift. The muscle clean first allows the athlete to focus on the upper body movement and precise placement of the bar in the rack position; the subsequent clean puts this into practice. Numbers can be pushed in either direction for emphasis; for example, if the muscle clean is relatively new or inconsistent, something like 3 muscle cleans + 1 clean may work well; in other cases, a single muscle clean before one or more cleans might be all that's necessary.

Power Clean + Clean

One of my favorite complexes for encouraging lifters to meet the bar better in their cleans is the power clean + clean. The power clean first gets the lifter pulling completely and meeting the bar tightly in a high position. The key is that the athlete should be attempting to rack the bar at the same height in the subsequent clean, then riding it down into the squat rather than locking off the receiving position at that height. Same thing goes here for reps as was described for the muscle clean + clean.

These exercises can be done as standalone technical work in other training sessions not involving cleans, or they can be used at the beginning of clean training sessions to help improve the subsequent clean work.

THE POWER SNATCH: USES AND CAUTIONS

I've nearly always defined a power snatch (or clean) by a receipt above a parallel squat. This is how I was taught. For the most part, I continue to use this definition because it's served me fine. However, at times I change my expectations based on what I want achieved. My other definition is no less than a 90-degree angle at the knee. This is a considerably higher receiving position—there is no question at this height of whether or not a lift can be classified as power. You won't be able to measure 90 degrees exactly, but it's not hard to get it close enough.

Caution

Defining a power snatch as a snatch received with the legs above horizontal is generally fine because much of the power snatch work a lifter does will not be at weights that force such a low position; that is, there won't be many times where a close call has to be made. This raises the question, however, of what we're trying to achieve by power snatching, and the answer to that will vary somewhat depending on the circumstances. We may be using the power snatch as an early exercise in the snatch learning process; we may be using it as a way to force somewhat lighter training on a given day; we may be using it to encourage an athlete to do something in particular, usually extending more forcefully, changing directions more quickly, or pulling under and fixing the bar overhead more aggressively.

There are three primary problems with pushing the weights of the power snatch up high. First is that athletes will tend to throw the feet out much wider than their squat positions. Some coaches couldn't care less about this and actually teach it. That's fine, but the reason I don't like it is simple: a miss in this position gets dicey because the athlete can't simply ride the bar down into a squat and turn a power snatch attempt into a snatch. Instead, you end up with some unwanted stress on the hips and knees, and with the bailout, most likely some strain to the shoulders and elbows.

Second, it's very difficult to actually stop a squat at just above parallel, especially with a ballistic load. Athletes will naturally avoid bending the knees that much because their bodies know how rough it will be. To compensate for the lack of depth at the knee, the lifter will hinge forward more at the hip and bring the arms farther back behind the head to keep the bar in place over the feet. Not only is this putting the shoulders and elbows in a sketchy position and asking for injury, but it's changing the mechanics of the lift, making the transition between power snatch and snatch more difficult. In my opinion, the two lifts should be identical and there should be no difficulty moving between them; this can only happen, however, if the two lifts are intentionally performed the same way.

Finally, the anticipation of getting the bar overhead so high with heavier weights can cause the lifter to tense up the arms rather than keeping them relaxed and focusing tension in the back. This makes the lift clumsy and typically slower, as well as causing the speed of the turnover and the aggressiveness of the punch up against the bar to suffer.

All of these potential problems can be avoided, but caution needs to be taken to do so.

Uses

Some coaches and athletes use the power snatch extensively; others in limited amounts; yet others refuse to use it entirely. There has been success in weightlifting with a lot of different methods, so I'm not going to condemn any of these approaches. As with most things, I'm of the opinion that the power snatch has utility at certain times and with certain athletes, and is inappropriate at other times or with other athletes. Maybe this sounds like unhelpful ambivalence, but unfortunately, that's how I think most things in the training world work. I'll run through some of the most common uses for the power snatch and mention some benefits and drawbacks.

Teaching The power snatch can be used as part of a teaching progression for the snatch. I personally use it almost every time I teach the snatch at least briefly. How much it's used and for how long depends on the athlete and the circumstances. But the power snatch is useful in this situation because nearly everyone is flexible enough to do it (which is not at all the case for the snatch), it helps ensure new lifters extend completely and aggressively, it helps teach the effort to turn the bar over aggressively and fix it tightly overhead as quickly as possible, and it limits the number of details the athlete is thinking about at this early stage of learning. As I've mentioned previously, I believe the power snatch and snatch are no different technically, so an athlete learning the power snatch before the snatch should present no problems at all, particularly when the goal is to progress them to doing snatches as soon as possible. One potential drawback of learning the power snatch first is that the athlete may develop a hesitation during the receipt of the bar before squatting. This is usually minor, temporary and can be combated quite well by making sure an athlete at this stage is also doing plenty of overhead squats and even snatches in addition when possible, such as in complexes of power snatch + snatch.

THE PORTABLE GREG EVERETT

Warm-ups Some athletes use the power snatch to warm-up for snatches. On this one I do have to agree with folks like Tommy Kono and Matt Foreman (you're welcome Matt—now you can say you've been mentioned alongside the great Tommy Kono) that it's not a great idea for most lifters. To clarify, I'm talking about a lifter starting with power snatches and moving to snatches as the weight increases. Some lifters are able to do this seamlessly, but more tend to reach a rough transition point. If multiple reps are being done at lighter weights, a lifter can start with a power snatch and end with a snatch each set to help combat this, e.g. power snatch + snatch at 50, 70, 90, then snatch at 110, 120, etc. I would prefer to just see snatches, although I like to see all snatches received high (relatively) and ridden down.

Technical Work Power snatches can have a variety of uses for technical work. The most common are probably encouraging a more aggressive finish, a quicker change of direction at the top, and a more aggressive turnover. Like any technical drill, there is no guarantee the power snatch will force a lifter to do any of these things. It will vary among lifters and circumstances, so it's incumbent on the coach or lifter to evaluate each time to ensure they're achieving the desired effect. Like with warm-ups, I like the combination of power snatches with snatches at times. An example of a good use for such a complex would be to encourage a lifter to meet the bar better in the snatch. A lifter who tends to drop out from under the bar and let it crash down and becomes unstable as a result can benefit from the feel of turning the bar over high and meeting it immediately and tightly; follow the power snatch immediately with a snatch, and the lifter can apply that concept and feeling to the snatch—because the weight is the same, they should be attempting to turn the bar over and fix it overhead at approximately the same height before sitting in to the squat. The previously discussed potential problems need to be kept in mind and effort needs to be made to avoid them especially in cases in which the power snatch is being used for technical improvement—it's not wise to try to fix one problem with a drill that creates another problem.

Reduced Intensity Power snatches and power cleans are often used as substitutes for the full lifts in order to reduce training intensity in general and minimize leg fatigue specifically. This might be for a taper week or a lighter training day or period. This reduces intensity and leg fatigue while keeping the athlete performing essentially the same skills.

Modification The power snatch can be used as an alternative to the snatch for individuals working around flexibility limitations or injuries. The former is very common with athletes new to the lift and it's preferable in my mind to have them learning and practicing the mechanics of the lift as soon as possible rather than either delaying the use of the lift until flexibility is adequate, or having the athlete perform the lift with an unsound bottom position. Flexibility can take a long time to improve, and an improper bottom position opens up the athlete to injury and also changes the mechanics of the lift to some extent, so it's arguably not any better than simply using the power snatch instead if you believe the power snatch and snatch are not identical.

Variety Finally, the power snatch can be used simply to introduce some variety into a training cycle that might otherwise be extremely monotonous if comprised entirely or nearly so of the classic lifts and squats. Preventing mental burnout is critical to keeping lifters motivated and productive and even seemingly minor modifications like this can have surprisingly dramatic effects.

Ultimately, decisions about exercise selection need to be made based on the needs and abilities of each athlete and the circumstances in which that athlete is training. What works for one lifter can be counterproductive for another. Avoid dismissing any exercise entirely, and let the needs of each situation dictate the approach.

OVERHEAD STABILITY IN THE SNATCH

When an athlete has difficulty supporting the bar overhead in the snatch, it's natural to immediately assume there is insufficient strength and to address the problem with strength work. While this may often be the problem, or at least one part of it, there are other elements to consider that may be preventing the athlete from properly using what may be adequate strength. In some cases, these problems can be corrected very quickly and save everyone a lot of headaches.

When it comes to supporting weight overhead, proper structure is the most important element. Strength is required to reinforce that structure, but we're not relying on muscular strength directly. The ability to lockout the elbows in the snatch or jerk is extremely important, and this can be easily demonstrated. Press a weight overhead and stop just short of elbow lock; when you begin to fail, lock the elbows completely and you'll find you can suddenly continue holding the weight. This is why individuals without the ability to completely lock the elbows are at a huge disadvantage in the sport, although there have been world records set by lifters with very poor elbow extension.

By creating the proper structure to support the bar, we maximize the potential of our strength. In the snatch, we can look at a few things. First, we need to create a solid foundation, which is the shoulders and upper back in this case. The shoulder is an extremely mobile joint, which has its advantages clearly, but also means there is a lot of potential for unwanted movement and instability. In order to create a solid foundation at the base of our structure, the shoulder blades must be fixed tightly in a position that prevents movement, allows the arms to rise as needed to the bar, and allows positioning of the weight and body to maintain balance over the feet. This can be achieved by completely retracting the shoulder blades and allowing them to upwardly rotate enough to open space for the humerus. I find the easiest way to accomplish this position is to imagine pinching the top inside edges of the shoulder blades together. This is not a shrug, although the upper traps will contract and bunch up.

The elbows must be locked out; in other words, they will be extended to the end of their range, which will normally be slight hyperextension. This creates the bone lock described previously and allows the muscles of the arm to support much more weight than they could directly. The elbows should be squeezed into extension directly rather than finding some indirect cue to encourage their extension. For example, many athletes have been told to pull the bar apart or something similar; I don't like these kinds of cues for a couple reasons. First, in order to pull the bar apart, you have to grip it tightly; a tight grip on the bar will limit how well you can extend the elbows. Second, I find this attempt makes it more difficult to secure the proper scapular position, and without this, the rest falls apart. That being said, if an athlete thinks of this cue and does what he or she is supposed to do, I won't argue about it. (Athletes can experiment with a variation of this by trying to push the bar apart rather than pull; this will allow the hands to stay more relaxed, encourage pressure through the palm rather than the fingers, and encourage a tightly secured base at the shoulder blades.)

This brings us to the hands. The bar should be in the palm slightly behind the centerline of the forearm. The hand and wrist should be allowed to settle in so the wrist is extended; do not try to hold the wrist in a neutral position. Again, if the bar is in the proper place in the hand, this will not place undue strain on the wrist, because it's not way behind the wrist as some mistakenly hold it. However, the proper hand and wrist position does require a good deal of mobility, which should be worked for diligently to allow the athlete to hold the proper positions as quickly as possible. If the athlete is flexible enough, the hook grip can be maintained overhead, but the grip must be relaxed to allow the hand and wrist to settle in properly.

The bar should be positioned over the back of the neck or the top of the traps with the head pushed forward through the arms somewhat. If the head is straight up or tucked back as some try to hold it, the shoulder blades cannot be held in the proper position and the arms cannot be oriented well to support the weight.

The width of the grip is another factor to consider. Ideally the grip can be such that the bar contacts the body in the crease of the hips. However, due to variations in body proportions, this can occasionally create problems elsewhere. The wider the grip, the more likely a lifter is to over rotate and drop the bar behind during the turnover of the snatch. Additionally, as the grip gets wider, it becomes more difficult to extend the elbows forcefully. A balance needs to be found between proper bar positioning during the pull and the ability to support and stabilize the bar overhead.

Finally, overhead instability can arise from the lower body entirely at times. Most commonly this is due to inflexibility, but can also be due simply to improper positioning. Most obviously, if an athlete has insufficient range of motion in the ankles and hips (or thoracic spine), he or she will not be able to establish a sound, upright squat, and as a consequence, he or she will not be able to establish the ideal overhead structure described previously. This may be because the trunk is forced to incline forward too much, the weight of the entire system is out of balance forward, or likely a combination of the two. Adequate flexibility throughout the body must be a priority for all lifters.

Spend some time investigating your or your athlete's overhead problems with the above information and see if you discover anything unexpected. The better you can diagnose the problem, the more quickly and easily you'll be able to correct it.

THE POINT

I spend a lot of time on this website and elsewhere discussing weightlifting technique, often in intolerably boring detail. Why technical proficiency is necessary and important is been mentioned with regard to things like CrossFit™ and athletic training, but it occurred to me last night that I can't think of a time when I've said explicitly why it's important for… weightlifters.

Maybe this is unnecessary and I'm concerned for no reason, but presumably you've come to accept my verbosity and affinity for repetition and will not find this an affront to your intellectual magnificence. I find myself giving this explanation to lifters in my own gym when I'm unmercifully hammering them with technical work and starting to wonder if they resent it or understand it.

Anyway, the point is this: The purpose of mastering weightlifting technique is to ultimately make the movements so natural that all of a lifter's focus and energy can be channeled into producing power. That is, the less of a lifter's resources are directed into ensuring proper mechanical execution of the lifts, the more of those resources can be directed into aggressive, vicious, explosive and decisive activation of the body.

The reason this issue gets complicated is that in the US, we're overwhelmingly dealing with adults or at least late adolescents who have athletic backgrounds in sports other than weightlifting. Their introduction and development is occurring relatively late, and as a consequence, the process often looks different than it would in cases of the systematic recruitment and development of children into certain sports.

Primarily this difference is the timeframe in which such development needs to occur. In the ideal situation, motor patterns can be learned and ingrained extremely rigidly very early in youngsters with little or no flexibility limitations. The remainder of a lifter's career can then be dedicated to developing strength and speed, with the repetition of technically consistent classic lifts with heavy weights further ingraining the skill. (Watch the elite of weightlifting in competition and you'll notice that their misses typically look essentially identical to their makes with the exception of whatever extremely minor detail caused the miss; in contrast, US lifters' misses are more likely to look significantly different than their makes.)

Instead of this, US lifters are often attempting to develop technical proficiency (and flexibility) alongside strength and speed. The processes are both abbreviated and conflated in a way that complicates the progression of the lifter considerably. This is not to say a good job can't be done with US lifters coming to the game late; but it certainly makes it more difficult and special considerations need to be made.

The more time and effort you put into learning the lifts and mastering technical execution in the earliest stages of your foray into weightlifting, the more successful you will be, and possibly as appealing, the less overall time you will need to dedicate to technical work.

MENSTICULAR FORTITUDE

Weightlifting is a very mental sport and success can be dependent on focus and attitude to remarkable degrees. Mental and testicular (or ovarian, if you prefer) fortitude is imperative not only for a given lift, but for a training session, a week, a cycle or a career.

The long term fortitude is usually thought of more as discipline. For example, the discipline to eat when, what and how much is necessary, the discipline to sleep adequately, the discipline to deny yourself activities or other things that interfere with your training, the discipline to sit in a bathtub full of ice in the middle of winter, the discipline to perform unglamorous and boring preparatory or rehab work.

When it comes to the fortitude necessary for training sessions, this is usually the will to not only get the work done, but to push yourself beyond what you feel you're capable of. There are many days you'll feel exhausted, weak, unmotivated, distracted or otherwise disinclined to train or to commit full effort and focus to training. These are the days you earn your progress, because these are the days that test your commitment. Everyone loves training when they feel good and perform well—doing what you're expected to do on these days is nothing special. It's the days you can barely force yourself to tie your shoes or put the bar on your back for the first time that define your character as an athlete. Are you going to surrender to complacency and comfort, or are you going to refocus on your goals and step up to the challenge?

Remember that on these days, the hardest part is usually getting started. You're stiff, you feel weak, you're moving slowly, your joints ache and your eyes are swollen with exhaustion. At this point, you're convinced there's no way you'll accomplish anything worthwhile in such a state. But if you can get yourself moving, as slowly as necessary for as long as necessary, you'll invariably begin to feel better. Your body will warm, your joints will produce more synovial fluid, your nervous system will start firing a bit more quickly, and with all of these gradual improvements, your mental state will improve as well. No one ever gets worse. This is not to say that if you can get yourself to start moving, you'll always feel great. You may very well hate every moment of that training session. But you have to remind yourself that you don't have to enjoy every moment of training and competition—you only have to love more moments than you hate.

When it comes to individual lifts or sets, mental fortitude takes on a somewhat different shape. You need not only the will to perform the task, but the will to focus only on that task, forget everything else, even the set or lift that immediately preceded it. You can't go back and change a set or a lift you've already done; you have control only over the lifts you have yet to do, and any energy or focus directed to anything else only limits your ability to get the job done. One of the most difficult things a weightlifter can do is come back and make a lift after a miss. If you fail to control yourself, you'll be crippled by doubt and hesitation. You must find ways to forget what you've done and concern yourself only with what you will do.

Even successful lifts can create problems. Just as you can't allow a prior miss to prevent you from focusing on your next lift, you can't allow a prior make to prevent you from focusing on your next lift. Confidence is a necessity for success, but confidence based on prior performance without focus and confidence on current performance can prevent adequate commitment to a lift.

Approach every rep as if it's your first and last.

THE ROLE OF STRENGTH IN WEIGHTLIFTING

While the premise of this article may at first strike readers as odd, considering that weightlifting, despite considerable elements of skill and speed, is very clearly a strength sport, there exist quite a few perspectives regarding the role of strength in the training of weightlifters; or, more accurately, regarding the appropriate degree of emphasis of what might be considered non-specific strength work.

The spectrum is represented on one end by Bulgarian-style training, involving little other, if anything at all, than the classic lifts and squats; the other end is represented by more of a powerlifting influence, involving a relatively large volume of general strength development with exercises like squatting, deadlift and pressing variations.

With weightlifting, as is the case with all physical training, we are possessed of few irrefutable facts, and constantly inundated with ideas, theories and anecdotes. And as with just about everything involving opinions, arguments and full-scale warfare continue to rage unabated (thanks in large part to the wondrous liberty and absence of consequence provided by the internet).

Also like with most similar endeavors, success is being achieved with a variety of methods, proving that no perfect approach exists—or at least that it has yet to be discovered.

Strength

Strength is a physical quality that is manifested in many different forms, some of which, it turns out, have little or nothing to do with each other in a practical sense. The most pertinent example in this case is the transfer of slow strength to explosiveness, or, more accurately, the lack thereof. Both anecdote and research have demonstrated that the ability to move very heavy weights slowly does not transfer well to the ability to move weights explosively; however, training explosively can improve an athlete's ability to move very heavy weights at any speed1.

This is the basis for many weightlifting coaches' aversion to exercises like deadlifts—they want to avoid slow, grinding movements for fear of limiting the athlete's ability to perform a similar movement explosively.

On the other hand, it's often argued that developing and maintaining a greater base of less than perfectly specific strength will provide more potential for classic lift performance. For example, if an athlete is able to clean 70% of his best deadlift, it seems logical that a heavier deadlift will result in a heavier potential clean.

Considering various weightlifters, the truth appears to be far less simplistic. It's not uncommon for weightlifters who never train the deadlift to out-deadlift their deadlifting counterparts. Of course, there are also plenty of examples of successful weightlifters who do employ the deadlift regularly.

Kendrick Farris is currently the best weightlifter in the US (he has cleaned and very nearly jerked the current world record as an 85 kg (187 lb) lifter—218 kg (480 lbs)), and accordingly, is often used for examples of effective training methodology. His coach, Dr. Kyle Pierce of LSU Shreveport, employs a system of classic periodization and a considerable volume of basic strength lifts such as deadlifts. Farris is extraordinarily strong; for example, he recently back squatted 235 kg (518 lbs) for 10 reps.

On the other end of the spectrum is Pat Mendes, who trains with coach John Broz in Las Vegas. At 130 kg (286 lbs), Pat has snatched 200 kg (441 lbs) and cleaned 230 kg (507 lbs)—2.5 kg more in the snatch and just 7.5 kg less in the clean & jerk than Shane Hammon's American record lifts—at the age of 19. Pat trains with Bulgarian-type methods, relying on the snatch, clean & jerk and front and back squats for the overwhelming majority of his training.

Would either be better having trained the other way? It's impossible to know. What we do know is that both ways *can* work. The Bulgarians have their stripped system of heavy classic lifts; the Chinese have a system of huge variety and a great deal of strength work. Other countries have systems using elements of both. All are producing extraordinary weightlifters.

Us Against The World

The US's performance on the international weightlifting stage has been less than impressive for the last few decades. Opinions vary on the reasons for this, but no one denies the fact that Americans are lagging far behind.

The trite phrase being tossed around the internet is, "American weightlifters just aren't strong enough." Such a statement is as useful and insightful as telling a sprinter he isn't fast enough. The question is how this can be changed, and this is where the arguments begin.

The idea that the US's poor international performance can be attributed to a single reason is silly at best. There are myriad factors contributing to the current state of weightlifting, and to neglect some to focus on a few that seem easier to correct is securing failure.

The more dominant countries in the sport have extensive infrastructure that provides for the recruiting and development of appropriate talent for the sport. They have cultures that recognize and appreciate weightlifting and weightlifters. They have fewer alternate sports to divert weightlifting talent. They have a greater number of lifters. And always looms the fact that drug testing in many of these countries is questionable, and by most accounts, drug use is commonplace.

In the US, weightlifting is an extremely obscure sport. Even if potential athletes happen to be exposed to it, there is little motivation to become involved. Sports like football, baseball, track and field, and gymnastics offer far more potential for financial and social success; additionally, these sports are ubiquitous, and coaches, facilities and related programs are easy to find. In contrast, weightlifters often must go to great lengths to even find a gym in which they can perform the lifts, let alone a qualified coach.

Considering the disparities in the circumstances, it's little surprise the US is not a leader in the sport. To chalk it up simply to inferior training methods is nonsense.

Making the Decision

If it's true, as it appears to be, that no single approach is best and that multiple methods can be effective, how does a weightlifting coach or weightlifter decide how to train? This is a decision that will hinge on multiple factors, but in all cases, it must be made in accordance to the needs of the lifter and his or her response to any given method. The biggest mistake any coach or athlete can make is to remain rigidly committed to a single approach when it becomes apparent that it no longer works or never worked in the first place. Experimentation carries some degree of risk, but it also provides the opportunity for discovery.

In a system that starts lifters at a young age with no previous athletic experience, a more consistent plan among athletes is possible. That is, these athletes can be collectively developed according to common need—the instruction and development of classic lift technique, the development of general and specific strength, and the development of work capacity.

In the US, there is essentially an absence of a system. Weightlifters typically arrive at the sport at later ages following other athletic careers. As a result, there is far more variation in the abilities, capacities and needs of US weightlifters, and consequently no simple prescription can be applied across the board. If a lifter is extremely strong, but technically unsound or inconsistent, it makes little sense to emphasize strength work over classic lift work; if a lifter is technically sound but simply doesn't have enough strength, strength work can be prioritized and classic lift work reduced. This kind of individualization can be difficult to implement with large groups of weightlifters, but fortunately, such groups really don't exist in the US.

The bottom line is that without a huge pool of athletes appropriate for the training, training must be made entirely appropriate for the athletes in order for any reasonable level of success to be achieved.

TECHNIQUE DRILLS AND TRAINING LIFTS

There seems to be a bit of discussion on technique training and strength training for weightlifters, and it's made me think of a couple points I want to clarify. First, how do you define a technique drill or a training exercise? In my opinion, the difference is based on the purpose, and a symptom is usually different loading and volume. We should also understand the difference between these two things and a learning/teaching drill.

A learning drill is an exercise intended to teach someone a movement or part of a movement; this is in the case of no former experience, or the case of improvement and/or modification of limited former experience. This is where you will see very light weights, or virtually no weight at all, and generally a much larger volume of repetitions. For example, this is where one might see the dreaded PVC pipe. More on that in a bit.

A technique drill is used to modify existing technique to bring it closer to what is desired. This is usually focused on a single technical element, but often you will address more than one unavoidably. Technique drills will be partial movements; sometimes very small pieces of a classic lift, and sometimes movements that are not at all derived from classic lifts (Examples of the latter would be things like snatch balance variations or pressing variations).

These will be performed with relatively light weights to ensure the athlete is executing them properly; improper execution is not only not helpful, it's counterproductive. These are motor pattern learning opportunities, but ones that allow or require some reasonable amount of resistance to be effective or possible. We will usually see segments of a classic lift or complexes here. For example, for a lifter who is not staying over the bar properly, we might perform a halting snatch deadlift, stopping at the hip with the shoulders over the bar, followed immediately by a snatch.

This leads us into training exercises. With respect to weightlifting, a training exercise is one that develops strength, speed or power (or all three) primarily. These are your obvious lifts such as the classic lifts, squats, pulls, push presses, etc. However, in this category we can also include things that look suspiciously like technique drills; the difference will be the weight used.

Using the previous example of a lifter not staying over the bar properly, we used a halting deadlift + snatch complex to teach the proper movement. However, if an athlete has been opening the hips early in his snatch, it's likely that his strength has developed around this movement and these positions, and as a consequence, no matter how well he can perform the lift at lighter weights, as he approaches maximal loads, his body will unavoidably revert to the positions in which it's strongest. This is when we now have to add strength to motor patterns. We may use a halting snatch deadlift just as we did previously, but drop the snatch and increase the loading. The key is to never take the loading beyond what allows the lift to be performed properly, because this will just take us right back to reinforcing the pattern we're trying to break. With this additional positional strength and the newly learned pattern, the lifter will naturally apply it to the lift we're trying to improve. Interestingly enough, the trickiest part of using a training exercise to correct a technical problem is teaching the lifter to perform it correctly - if he already knew how to do it well, he wouldn't be doing it. So you end up teaching technique anyway, just in a less direct manner.

Ultimately, the definitions are somewhat nebulous and in practice, there will often not be a simple demarcation between two. More important than naming things is knowing when and how to apply them.

The basics come down to this: When teaching a skill, weight is largely irrelevant. At some early point, there must be some resistance, e.g. an empty barbell, because the athlete needs a degree of feedback regarding position and movement that PVC pipe cannot provide. But there are certain elements of teaching you may use initially that preclude the use of even this weight. Once an athlete has learned the lifts at a basic level, weight will be progressively increased on average, and technique drills will become more specific to individual need. In this intermediate stage, weight should never exceed technical ability - deviation from proper execution simply strengthens improper execution. The priority is strengthening the correct movement, not simply loading up the weight indiscriminately to create some false sense of improving strength. Once a legitimate level of technical proficiency is reached, training exercises will constitute the bulk of an athlete's work, with technical drills or technique-specific training exercises playing a very small role - used only to address specific issues as they arise.

To circle back around to PVC pipe as I said I would, this is something worth clarification since the internet is so good at creating and perpetuating nonsense. No established weightlifter trains with PVC pipe; the only use it may get is as a tool for stretching. When I teach the snatch to a brand new lifter, I start with PVC pipe, no matter the size or strength of the individual. I use an extensive series of teaching drills, some of which simply cannot be done with much else. Larger guys can often use a 10kg bar initially, but they spend too much time doing it wrong for it to be worthwhile simply to assuage their egos and prove to a few keyboard warriors that weightlifters aren't weak. But after this initial progression (which is usually very brief—measured in minutes), these new lifters move right to a barbell and generally never return to PVC.

Every coach has his own approach to teaching and training the lifts, and no one with any kind of experience or reason would say there is a perfect or correct approach suitable for all athletes at all times. The common theme, however, is the goal of developing lifters who are not only strong nor only technically proficient, but both, and in weightlifting, the two traits can never be completely isolated.

STRENGTH. AGAIN.

This discussion will not die, so I will poke at it a bit more. US weightlifters need to get stronger. This is the refrain repeated endlessly from many outside the weightlifting community. From inside the community, the response is essentially a unanimous agreement in principle—of course in a strength sport athletes need to get stronger. Where the argument really exists is with regard to what exactly that means and how to achieve it.

First, weightlifters compete in the snatch and clean & jerk. That's it. Nothing else matters at all. While it may be interesting to know a certain lifter has a huge squat or has done some other weird feat of strength outside of this, it won't change his competitive results—he either snatches and clean & jerks more or less than the next guy.

What individuals with little steeping in weightlifting seem to be unable to understand is how specific the needs of weightlifters really are. It's exceptional in its specificity with regard to strength, especially from the perspective of someone who works on building strength in a very general sense for non-strength athletes. If you work only with football players, it probably seems like more strength in any form = better potential performance, and this is largely true because football players don't have a perfectly specific manner of expressing strength in the sport. This is not the case in weightlifting.

A great example that I've seen come up numerous times is the idea that getting stronger in the press will improve the jerk. To be fair, a lifter must have adequate upper body strength to support larger and larger weights overhead, but supporting a weight is much different than putting it there. Most female weightlifters are great examples of this—the typical gal is not at all good with pressing strength, yet will be able to jerk huge amounts of weight. It's normal for female lifters to have much larger jerk:press ratios than men. What this comes down to is simple: a conviction that striving for better press numbers as a primary goal in order to improve the jerk demonstrates a lack of understanding of the jerk. Of all the possible jerk accessory exercises available, the press is possibly the least helpful.

The last thing I'll mention is the notion that ever-increasing numbers in basic lifts like the deadlift will drive improvements in the snatch and clean. Certainly there is a relationship between these lifts, but it's not that straightforward. Generally speaking, a lifter with a bigger deadlift will out clean and snatch a lifter with a smaller deadlift—but only when we're talking about large differences. Moreover, weightlifters who never actually deadlift in training are often capable of huge deadlifts—so which is driving which?

Some argue that beyond the beginner level, the snatch and clean & jerk can't drive increases in strength. This is utter nonsense that can only be genuinely believed by someone who has never actually snatched and clean & jerked heavy weights. A powerlifter with a 600+ lb deadlift who snatches 180 lbs will feel that snatches are extremely light and will not understand how snatching could possibly make one stronger. In this case, he is right—he's snatching 30% or so of his best deadlift. But seasoned lifters are better at putting their available strength to use in the lifts, and as a consequence, their classic lifts are much greater percentages of their top strength numbers. For example, a lifter may snatch more like 60%+ of his best deadlift—a much different prospect than 30%.

This is not to say that doing the snatch and clean & jerk exclusively is the best method of improving strength for weightlifting. The point is that discounting the ability of the classic lifts to build weightlifting-specific strength is a product of having no understanding of weightlifting.

Do lifters need to push their squats? Of course—I don't know any who don't. This is constantly returned to by folks as well—if lifters would just train the squat harder, they would get stronger, and their lifts would go up. The funny part is that I don't know any lifters who don't push their squats. This is some weird notion that has gained traction outside the weightlifting community. My assumption is that those claiming this is what's going on, and claiming to have interaction with lifters who report this is happening, are actually talking to brand new lifters (or individuals who go to train with good lifting coaches a few times). In these cases, these coaches are likely spending most if not all the time with these individuals working on the snatch and clean & jerk, and likely with light weights much of the time, because these individuals need to learn how to snatch and clean & jerk before they can do much else. To see this as reflective of that coach's actual training programs is absurd.

Most of you reading this would have to change your underwear if you saw the squatting my better lifters do—usually 4-6 days/week, sometimes twice daily, and not necessarily with low volume. The idea that weightlifters in the US just fiddlefart around with baby weights and technique work their whole careers is absolutely ridiculous.

BEGINNING WEIGHTLIFTING AS AN ADULT

In my dreams, I coach in a system like the Chinese, in which I have a few dozen elite lifters handed to me between the ages of 18-20 after they've spent the last 8-10 years training under excellent coaches and are already world-class lifters at this young age. These athletes are professional weightlifters, with no obligations or responsibilities in life beyond snatching and clean & jerking more weight. Additionally, their compliance with my prescriptions would be closely approaching 100%. I would also have several assistant coaches who were extremely well-educated and experienced.

As it turns out, this is not much like the situation I'm actually in, which I suspect is essentially the same as that of a great many individuals who make a living in a similar fashion. Most of my lifters and other clients have jobs, school, families and most started lifting as adults. As requested by some of our readers, this article will focus on training weightlifters who start and lift as adults rather than the supple, malleable promising young brats we'd all prefer to be and to coach.

With such athletes, we have quite a few considerations to make that we wouldn't have to worry about with youngsters, such as limited training time due to job, school and family obligations, decreased flexibility and mobility, limitations—either physical or psychological—from past injuries, an often stunning collection of bad habits, and the inevitable reduction in recovery and work capacity that accompanies increasing age.

Those individuals who arrive at weightlifting with some kind of previous athletic experience often have decent strength bases unlike young kids. This can be both beneficial in some respects and a real problem in others. On the one hand, it's less you have to work on; on the other hand, that strength is rarely specific enough to be entirely applicable, and strong individuals typically have egos that make them resistant to using appropriately light weights for periods of technical instruction and practice. Managing this is really an issue of being confident in what you're teaching and the resulting respect your athletes and clients have for you as a coach. If your athletes don't listen to you, check your own confidence, ability and presence before you start blaming them.

Part of this confidence and respect is being honest enough to admit when you don't know something—don't try to make something up. If you don't know, tell your athlete and let him or her know that you will find out.

Of course with multiple problems present, you won't have the luxury of working on them individually—you will find yourself trying to manage correction of all of them together. This can be a bit overwhelming, but you can make it a bit easier by initially considering them all individually and then adjusting as needed when you attempt to bring everything together. That is, what you may decide is the perfect prescription to correct some flexibility limitations may become a bit excessive when you add in strength work, technique work and whatever else you're doing. Consequently, you will need to cut it back a bit to allow some time for the rest.

Past Injuries

Limitations imposed by past injuries can be some of the toughest problems to cope with. Most often, you'll be dealing with many years of reduced range of motion, scar tissue accumulation, compensatory movement patterns, weakness, and even fear of certain positions and movements.

Although we'd all love to be experts in every area (Why don't you call a specialist, Joe? *I am a specialist.* At what? *At everything.*) I recommend seeking the assistance of an actual expert when working with significant problems. Of course, do your best to help your athletes and clients find a medical professional with experience treating athletes, not just dying post-hip-replacement geriatrics.

Try to communicate as much as possible with that professional about what you're seeing and what you're doing in the gym to give him or her a clearer understanding of the problem and what they're attempting to prepare the client for. Video of a dysfunctional movement pattern, for example, can be very helpful to a physical therapist or chiropractor who would otherwise not be able to view such a movement and be forced to rely largely on descriptions by the patient, which you probably know as well as I do are rarely accurate.

In addition to referring your clients to the appropriate medical professional, do what you can to educate yourself about the problem and find possible corrective strategies you can safely and effectively implement in the gym. The internet offers a vast amount of quality information, often at no cost—you have no excuse to not at least give it a shot.

In all cases, be conservative when attempting to introduce or reintroduce movements or positions to these clients. No matter what the nature of the limitation—physical or psychological—a more gradual progression will be safer and more effective. Keep your perspective long term and avoid trying to push too hard too fast because you or your client is simply impatient. Remember, the condition more than likely took years to develop—you're not going to fix it in three training sessions.

Decreased Mobility & Flexibility

Aside from reduced mobility and flexibility accompanying past injuries, you will encounter these problems with people who have developed them in the absence of any injury—either due to being sedentary or simply engaging in physical activity that never posed any kind of significant flexibility demands (e.g. running, cycling, walking, etc).

I've read (on the internet, of course) experts who claim adults cannot improve flexibility. I don't know where this notion comes from, but it was certainly not the same planet I work on. I have helped plenty of clients in their 40s and 50s increase their flexibility dramatically over the last several years. Perhaps whatever literature these guys got the idea from referred to some kind of "study" involving underpaid, unmotivated physical therapists "stretching" old people in assisted living facilities over a period of 30 days. It would not be terribly surprising to me if no significant changes in flexibility were observed in such circumstances.

Achieving considerable improvements in flexibility can be an extremely long, frustrating process, but it is entirely possible in all cases. Again, keep things in perspective—if you have a 50 year-old client who hasn't stretched or done any kind of flexibility-requiring activity for 30 years, you shouldn't be surprised to find their range of motion doesn't suddenly increase 25% after a week of stretching. Patience and consistency are the two most important elements of improving flexibility.

Never push stretches or mobility drills into the range of pain. Discomfort is fine—if it's comfortable, it's probably not doing anything. Mike Boyle likes to say that "Does it hurt?" is a yes-no question. Any qualification that accompanies a "no" response means the real answer is yes. If you hurt your client stretching, guess what? Not only will you fail to make the progress that you could, you will probably lose your client.

For individuals who work sedentary jobs, encourage them to get up and move around every hour or two whenever possible. Performing some basic dynamic warm-up type movements throughout the day will do absolute wonders for progress. Such a quick routine upon rising every morning will also be helpful.

While flexibility and mobility are working their way to ideal (or at least to necessary minimums for safety), modify training to avoid unsafe positions and movements. For example, those with limited shoulder and/or thoracic spine mobility or reduced arm adductor/internal rotator flexibility will often experience sharp pain when jerking. As a trainer or coach, pain during a movement should be a pretty straightforward indication to you that the movement should be stopped and some kind of assessment and corrective plan implemented. Alternatives can be used during this period of correction, and periodic re-assessment can be performed to determine when the excluded exercise can be re-introduced. In the jerk example, often these same people will have no pain during pressing or even push pressing, so these can be used. We may also do jerk supports, jerk recoveries, jumping squats, jerk split drops, jerk dip squats, jerk springs, and lunges and other unilateral leg strength exercises. There are always alternatives to doing nothing at all. Be creative and work around the problem while actively working to correct it.

Decreased Recovery Capacity

Unfortunately, as age and wisdom accumulate, the ability to recover from all the great new training methods you've learned decreases. This paradox is particularly aggravating, but short of pharmaceutical intervention, there is little we can do about it (and even the effectiveness of such intervention will continue decreasing over time).

Quite simply, a lifter in his or her forties will not be able to manage the same volume of training stress as a lifter in his teens or twenties. While the trend is consistent, the actual training volume and intensity each athlete can effectively manage is very individual. This is something, as with athletes of any age, that you will need to experiment with somewhat. Start conservatively, evaluate, and build up as tolerated rather than aiming high initially. Starting with what turns out to be excessive volume or intensity will make the process of determining what works much longer and more difficult than necessary. A week of excessive volume will take a week or even more sometimes to recover from, which means you've lost that much time (and possibly more) to evaluate the effects of the program as the athlete's response to training during that period will not accurately reflect its effect on him or her, but rather the effect it has with whatever degree of systemic fatigue is already present.

In addition to age, we can also consider bodyweight when trying to determine effective levels of volume—the larger the athlete, the less volume he or she will be able to handle. Again, the degree of change will be very individual, but expect to modulate the volume to some degree in accordance to bodyweight.

In addition to adjustments to the training program, lifestyle and nutrition elements should be emphasized to maximally utilize the recovery capacity that does exist. Sleep and other stress-reducing exercises are the number one priority (as they are for anyone). Often older adults have conditioned themselves for many years to survive on stunningly little sleep, and often that amount decreases as they age. This should be emphatically discouraged—these individuals are not growing in the sense that kids are, of course, but they will be constantly remodeling their bodies in response to training stress. This can only be successful in the presence of adequate rest.

Limited Training Time

Adults generally have far more responsibilities and obligations than their younger counterparts, and accordingly, are less likely to have flexible schedules and extensive tracts of time available for training. Sometimes this is due simply to poor time management and more time for training can be recovered through restructuring days and weeks; but sometimes it is entirely legitimate and it is an obstacle that will have to be worked around.

Fortunately, this decrease in available time for training mirrors the decrease in recovery capacity, and as a consequence, you may not actually be losing time you needed for more training. In fact, such scheduling restrictions can sometimes be a blessing, in that it naturally prevents the overly enthusiastic coach or athlete from prescribing or performing more work than can be managed.

Masters-age lifters will often make more progress training as little as 2-3 days per week. Don't be afraid to try less rather than more. You may also find that with more training days, it will be helpful to more dramatically modulate volume and intensity from day to day. That is, while you may program 3 consecutive days, the middle, and possible the third day as well, will be lower in volume and intensity than the first.

Bad Habits

Although there are bad habits of more than one nature that could potentially limit the progress of a lifter (foil-smoking cocaine, for example), in this case, I'm talking about technical habits. A more advanced age means more possible time to practice incorrect movements and consequently more difficulty in breaking them. Since this article is supposed to be about beginning weightlifting as an adult, this theoretically shouldn't be a problem as the lifts haven't been performed previously. However, this doesn't mean an individual hasn't performed other training in the gym with exercises that are somehow related enough to cause problems. The most obvious examples would be the basic strength lifts such as the squat, deadlift and press variations. Squatting and deadlifting habits in particular can be dramatic and tough to break, such as trying to sit back into an adjacent state when squatting, or leaning so far over the bar when deadlifting that your head slips up your ass.

Obviously corrections for technical problems will vary with the problem as well as the athlete, so they can't be covered here. My book, *Olympic Weightlifting: A Complete Guide for Athletes & Coaches*, has quite a few you can try out. The basic approach, though, is to be patient and consistent, just like with flexibility work. You won't fix a bad habit in one session—it can take weeks and months to correct certain habits.

Non-Compliance

There is nothing unique about adults with regard to compliance to a coach's prescriptions other than the potential for age differentials to interfere. That is, occasionally an older adult will be resistant to listening to a younger coach. This is not something I've personally had a problem with, but I've seen it and heard others' laments.

The advice for this problem is the same mentioned above with regard to the egos of strong people. If you're not actually good at what you do, not confident, and not respectable, you will not have compliant athletes, no matter the ages involved. Fix the problem.

Easily the best way to ensure compliance is to deliver results. I realize this is a bit of a paradox, as it's difficult to produce results if an athlete is not complying with your prescriptions. However, no one is 100% non-compliant (and I would hope that any such individuals would be summarily dismissed from your facility). Even with less than perfect compliance, a good program and good coaching will work to a significant extent. Use this success, and the success of your other athletes, to prove to resistant athletes that you know what you're doing rather than trying to talk them into it.

Finally, make it clear to your athletes that your effort and attention will be commensurate to their commitment and effort. Those athletes who are not willing to do what they need to do should not be receiving the same kind of coaching as your dedicated, hard-working, compliant athletes.

Bottom Line

Ultimately the key to success with weightlifting as an adult, either as a coach or the lifter, is to evaluate and program individually as you would with an athlete of any age. Obviously in a gym full of many lifters, you can't completely individualize for every one. However, you can always be evaluating your lifters' responses to their training and making individual adjustments to a general program. For example, at Catalyst Athletics, I write a program for the team that a number of lifters follow. A few of those lifters receive individualized work or modifications to the program as needed to address volume, schedule or technical needs. Then I write completely individual programs for other lifters who are at a high enough level to warrant it. I would love to write individual programs for all of them, but the reality is that many need essentially the same things anyway, and I simply don't have the time even if they didn't.

A helpful starting point is to write what you might consider the ideal program, without concern for being too heavy on the volume and intensity, and then pare it down to accommodate the needs of the adult lifter in question. Again, err on the side of too little rather than too much, and add things back in if tolerated.

THE SIMPLEST PROGRAM IN THE WORLD

I've written down this same program so many times for so many people, I thought it would make sense to put it down here for other people to use. I'm sure things that look a lot like this have been floating around for decades because it makes perfect sense and is remarkably simple. I think I may have stuck it or something very similar in a newsletter at some point in the last couple years as well. The basic structure is as follows:

Day 1
Snatch
Snatch Pull
Front Squat

Day 2
Jerk
Push Press
Overhead Squat

Day 3
Clean & Jerk
Clean Pull
Back Squat

The snatch, clean and jerk can be the classic lifts as written, or any variation of your choosing based on how you're feeling on a particular day, or based on what you need to address certain technical problems. This includes variations like powers, hangs, complexes, etc.

Snatch and clean pulls can be done as pulls as written, or you can substitute any pulling-related exercise such as halting deadlifts, partial pulls, segment pulls and pull complexes. Again, choose exercises that address your own needs with regard to technique and strength.

The push press on day 2 can be any kind of upper body press exercise that you decide is most effective: push press behind the neck, press, incline bench press, etc. Similarly, the overhead squat on day 2 can be replaced with a snatch balance variation, complex of snatch balance and overhead squat, snatch push press and overhead squat, etc.

Front squats and back squats on days 1 and 3 can be done with whatever sets and reps you choose. As a starting point, I would suggest 3s for the front squat and 5s for the back squat, 3-5 sets for each.

To this you can consider adding a technique exercise at the start of each day related to the classic lift of the day. For example, on day 1 if you have trouble with the turnover of the snatch, you might choose to do a few sets of muscle snatches or tall snatches before doing the snatches. Keep this exercise relatively light and easy.

Start the first week with fairly conservative weights and spend 3-4 weeks building the weights up, decreasing the reps or sets somewhat as you go if necessary. For example, you might do triples in the snatch, clean and jerk on week 1, doubles on week 2 and singles on week 3, increasing the weight by 5-10% each week.

Have fun with it.

PROGRAM DESIGN CASE STUDY

Program design is one of those topics that is overwhelming both to read and write about. Most literature is necessarily nebulous and vague, and individuals interested in learning more often find themselves inundated with a collection of concepts that fail to fit together easily than with a set of practical rules they can implement.

So instead of talking about ideas in this article, I want to run through the process of actually designing a real program and discuss the rationale for various decisions. The athlete whose program I'll be using as my example is probably fairly well representative of many PM readers with regard to age, obligations, recovery and the other factors that contribute to her particular difficulties. For our purposes here, we'll call her Brooke.

Brooke has been part of our lifting team for several months. She's in her mid-thirties, works a very stressful job, tends to take on additional hours, never sleeps enough, and usually fails to eat enough. However, she is extremely motivated and committed to lifting.

Technically she is quite good. There are a few issues that plague her, though, and have been extraordinarily frustrating. For example, as she reaches 85-90% or more snatching, she will begin shifting forward into the bar, cut off her pull and try to swing herself under the bar; in her cleans, she will again cut her pull short and drop out from under the bar, allowing it to pull her forward and crash on her. With regard to strength, her pulling is very strong relative to her classic lifts, but her squatting is comparatively weak, despite squatting being her favorite thing to do.

The way programming works with our team is that I write one team program that all lifters follow with minor individual modifications until they reach a point at which a completely individual program is necessary or warranted. Until this point, Brooke has been on the team program, but her progress has ground to a halt despite occasional off-the-cuff modifications to account for fatigue and technical issues. Following Nationals, I gave her a week off, during which she actually trained two days just doing light hang work and squats, and she began a program of her own this week.

When designing the program, I obviously wanted to take advantage of the fact that it was for her alone and could individualize it entirely. This means I could address her strength deficits, her technical needs and her recovery limitations exactly as I wanted to (short of making her quit her job, eat perfectly and sleep 14 hours a day).

The Basic Structure

Brooke's most pressing need is improving her leg strength. She has essentially brought her classic lift ability to the margins of her available strength. Because of her limited recovery capacity, I needed to reduce the volume and intensity of her other training in order to emphasize this strength development. At the same time, she needed to continue improving certain technical flaws.

I decided to use a squat cycle created by Tim Swords of Team Houston. This is a 7-week cycle that has her squatting 3 days each week, uses both front and back squats, and is fairly low volume. I've had success with it in the past with other athletes and like the principle behind it. This squat program created the foundation for Brooke's cycle. I will be monitoring her squatting efforts each day and considering the possibility of reducing the weight occasionally based on how difficult I expect a given squat session to be.

The lifting team trains Monday-Thursday and Saturday. I placed her squats on Tuesday, Thursday and Saturday for even spacing and because there is no consistent pattern in the cycle that would have the heaviest session falling on a certain day each week. Because recovery is a big issue, I kept other heavy lifts to these days, and left Monday and Wednesday reserved more for lighter technical work that wouldn't tax her unnecessarily, but would keep her moving and give us opportunities to improve technical elements that we needed to work on.

Volume & Intensity

The first week of the cycle, the volume comes in at just under 200 reps, which is low, but not extremely so—much of the volume is coming from light technique work, so I'm less concerned with its effect. This will reduce week to week for a few weeks, probably jump up a bit again, and then reduce until the final week of the program. I'm keeping this flexible and will adjust as I go in response to her performance.

The only weights I've prescribed for the entire cycle are for her squats, according to Coach Swords' program (which again, I may adjust slightly if needed). For the remaining exercises, I've prescribed only reps and sets. I will control the weights day to day according to how Brooke is lifting. The goal with these exercises is ensuring excellent and consistent execution, not reaching heavy weights— her squatting will take care of strength development during this cycle.

Brooke is prone to getting a little carried away with core training if left unsupervised, and will rack up quite a bit of additional volume hammering away at ab and back work. For this reason, I've prescribed exactly the core work I want her to do, and she knows to do only this.

Exercise Selection

With the foundation of the squat cycle in place, I needed to consider Brooke's remaining needs and work within my limited volume and intensity constraints to address them as well as possible. The most frustrating issue for Brooke is her stalled progress on the snatch; this frustration arises more from the fact that her failure to snatch heavier weights appears to be more of a mental and technical issue than a strength or speed issue. That is, as she approaches her maximum snatch weight, she departs from her previously sound technical execution and resorts to chasing the bar with her hips, shifting onto the balls of her feet too early, quitting her leg drive completely, and trying to swing the bar around and duck under it.

As a former volleyball player, Brooke's vertical jump was quite good. At present, it is about 17", which is decent for her height, but also indicative of a need to improve her explosiveness. This is also very clear in her heavier snatch and clean attempts. In order to work on this, I tacked on box jumps immediately after each set of squats. The number of jump reps will reduce over time as the squat cycle gets more demanding. Box height is selected to be comfortably under a maximum, but high enough to warrant some effort. Too high of a box, and athletes tend to cut their jumps short in order to reach their feet up to the box; this is a problem across the board, but particularly in this case, considering that one of Brooke's primary problems is quitting early on the leg drive of her snatch and clean. On Saturdays, I also have her doing box jumps as the first exercise in her workout as a way to try to get her firing both physically and mentally.

Brooke's cleans are considerably better and more consistent than her snatches, so far more emphasis is being placed on the snatch. Further, her jerk is outstanding and needs minimal practice. Generally I like to balance work between snatch and clean & jerk pretty evenly, but in the case of limited work capacity and recovery, it's important to prioritize.

Mondays are a snatch focus day. Brooke starts with a snatch high-pull + muscle snatch complex. The snatch high-pull accomplishes two primary goals— to encourage her to finish driving with her legs all the way to the top of the pull, and to elevate the elbows maximally rather than dropping them early to swing the bar. Brooke's snatch turnover has been weak and unaggressive historically, and one of the biggest problems with snatch turnovers in general is the absence of an aggressive initial pull against the bar with the arms to both accelerate the lifter down and set the bar and body position ideally to turn the arms over into the final overhead position.

Muscle snatches are also a commonly poorly-performed exercise, with athletes dropping the elbows and simply pressing the bar up awkwardly. The point of the muscle snatch is to strengthen the movement of the turnover—unless the positions and movements are correct, it will fail in this goal. Performing a snatch high-pull immediately before a muscle snatch is a reliable way to get a lifter to perform the muscle snatch with the necessary elbow elevation. The goal for the muscle snatches is to both drill the proper turnover movement and to strengthen it so it's less likely Brooke will deviate from it as her snatch weights increase.

In addition to this, the pull and muscle snatch both provide opportunities for Brooke to focus on her start position, in which she tends to keep her shoulders behind the bar rather than above it, and on getting back onto and staying on her heels.

The weight for this exercise is taken up gradually, and at the heaviest weight that is moving well and her elbows are reaching full height, I will stop her and have her perform the prescribed number of sets.

After this comes a snatch high-pull + snatch complex. Already Brooke has drilled the muscle snatch and snatch pull movements, so these parts of her snatches will be quite sound. Preceding each snatch with a snatch high-pull again encourages proper weight balance on the feet, complete leg drive with her extension, and the aggressive and complete elbow extension necessary for a good third pull.

Brooke will take the weight up gradually and I will choose the weight I want her to use for the prescribed sets and reps—this is a weight that she can perform as close to perfectly as can be expected.

She finishes Monday with a few sets of hanging leg raises.

On Tuesday, Brooke starts with mid-hang power cleans. The purpose of this exercise is to have her practice the proper finish for her cleans, to encourage a more aggressive change of direction and pull under, and meeting the bar with the shoulders higher. Like in the snatch, Brooke tends to slide forward on her feet and cut her leg drive short as her clean weights increase, and drop out from under the bar in an effort to get under it, which cause it to crash on her and limit her ability to recover.

Starting her in the mid-hang position lets me place her in the perfect second-pull position and allows her to feel where her balance should be on her feet and where the bar and her shoulders should be. This starting position also forces an aggressive extension, quick change of direction, and aggressive pull under because of the limited distance to accelerate the bar; forcing a power receipt increases these demands even more. The power clean additionally encourages her to receive the bar as quickly and as high as possible, and to aggressive resist the downward force, rather than pulling down indiscriminately and allowing the bar to fall and crush her.

Next Brooke performs 3 halting snatch deadlifts + 1 snatch pull. The focus for this exercise is the positioning and balance of the first and second pulls—more specifically, keeping the shoulders over instead of behind the bar off the ground; shifting back onto the heels immediately and staying there all the way to the top; and staying over the bar as long as possible. The halting snatch deadlift stops with the bar in the crease of the hips, the knees very slightly bent, the shoulders slightly in front of the bar, and the weight back on the heels. After 3 of these, she performs a snatch pull. The idea is that this pull will be consistently better because of the immediately preceding position practice with the halting deadlifts. Again, I control the weight of these to ensure quality execution. My goal is to be able to continue increasing the weight on these for the duration of the cycle, likely dropping the number of halting deadlifts as we go.

To finish the day, Brooke performs the week's first squat session.

On Wednesday, we start with 3 sets of 5 mid-hang muscle snatches. This is set up to really develop turnover strength—by starting from mid-thigh, the acceleration possible with the legs and hips is reduced and the shoulders and arms must do more of the work. Each rep must be done precisely.

Next, Brooke does mid-hang snatches. The rationale for these is similar to that described previously for the mid-hang power cleans; that is, we want to force correct position and aggressive and complete extension and turnover. The muscle snatches before help her keep the turnover strong and accurate.

She finishes the day with planks, weighted as needed to keep her times between 30-60 seconds. This keeps Wednesdays a fairly short and less-taxing day to give her some recovery room for Thursday's squats and the rest of the week.

On Thursday, Brooke gets a clean focus day. She starts with 3 halting clean deadlifts + 1 clean pull to accomplish the same thing described for the deadlift + pull complex on Tuesday. She then moves on to a power clean + clean complex. After the deadlift + pull complex, her positions tend to be better and more consistent. The power clean before the clean encourages her to be more aggressive at the top and with the change of direction and turnover, and also it gives her a reference point for the height at which she should be receiving the bar for the clean. Weights are again controlled by me according to how she's lifting. Brooke finishes the day with the week's second squat session.

After a rest day on Friday, Brooke gets to snatch and clean & jerk on Saturday without any drill work other than the 3 sets of box jumps she starts the day with. Weights will change week to week. On the first week, Brooke takes both up to the heaviest single she can do well that day. On week 2, she snatches to the heaviest single possible for the day, but does only 60% in her clean & jerk for 5 singles. On week 3, she will do the opposite of week 2. This will repeat, and on the final Saturday, she will get to take both to a max for the day. She then does her last squat session of the week, and finishes the day with more planks.

Flexibility

One of the primary themes of this cycle is flexibility. This is a tough one for many athletes and coaches, who have meltdowns at the thought of deviating from a plan. The reality of programming, however, is that it involves elements of estimation, guesswork, prediction and plain old luck. The chance of even a relatively short cycle, such as this 7-week one, going its duration without any unexpected problems is low. A great way to prevent progress is to force a rigid program onto a constantly changing set of circumstances. Having a plan is critical, but planning to adjust and adapt will allow that plan to be successful.

TWINKLE TOES

There is some current discussion on foot position in the squat following a post by Kelly Starrett, and I've been asked to comment. This article is not intended to criticize him or anyone else, nor is it intended to stand as irrefutable fact; its purpose is to quickly organize my thoughts on the topic and answer the requests for my input. Use the available information to make your own decisions on training and coaching.

Arguments for Toes Forward

The following is a quick and very basic summary of the arguments for squatting with the toes forward as presented by Kelly Starrett.

> Potential knee injury magnitude is reduced with a reduced valgus/rotational force.

> Squatting toes forward is motor learning to ensure this stance when jumping and landing; squatting with toes out teaches athletes to jump and land with the sub-optimal toes-out position.

> Landing with feet out means potential for valgus knee movement.

> Squatting with feet/knees out requires constant focus to maintain position—loss of focus means valgus knee movement.

> We need to prepare athletes in a way that limits the magnitude of potential injuries.

Toes-Out Squatting

The first question to ask is why do we squat with the toes out? There are two basic possible answers. The first is that we rotate the feet outward to match the direction of the thighs to ensure the knee is hinging soundly rather than twisting. The second is that the individual has flexibility limitations (namely limited ankle dorsiflexion, and/or tight adductors and/or internal hip rotators) and is forced to excessively turn the toes out and roll onto the inside edges of the feet to circumvent dorisflexion when trying to achieve a deep squat position. Clearly the latter is not a legitimate reason to squat with the toes out, but this also has no bearing on the argument because it's entirely unrelated—this is excessive and unintentional outward rotation.

While the hips have a large range of possible motion, there is a fairly narrow plane in which they can flex maximally. This plane varies slightly among individuals based on anatomical differences, but it's always a position of some external rotation. This is easily demonstrated by squatting to full depth in a narrow stance with the feet straight forward—you'll find it impossible to maintain an extended lumbar spine as the femurs hit the end range of motion against the pelvis. Now take the feet out a bit wider and turn them out a little and notice the feeling in your hips—the femurs will more freely move up in the hips. This can also be demonstrated in a seated position by pulling your knee straight up and back to your chest—you'll feel the hip max out. Now from this position, bring the knee out to the side and you'll find you're able to pull it farther back without feeling the compression of the femur against the pelvis.

This is why we squat with the knees out to some degree (that degree, as mentioned previously, a bit different from athlete to athlete)—to allow the fullest hip range of motion possible, which means the greatest depth possible while maintaining proper spinal extension.

Which brings us back to the feet. As I stated above, we turn the feet out to match the direction of the thighs. That is, if the thigh is exiting the hip at about 25 degrees from the centerline, we turn the feet out about 25 degrees from the centerline. If the feet are also placed at the correct width, this means that the knee hinges as it's intended rather than being twisted as it flexes. If the knee is not aligned when squatting, now we're not talking about potential catastrophic valgus knee failure—we're talking about repeated stretching of inelastic connective tissue surrounding the knee, leading to chronic knee pain, joint laxity and the resulting increased injury potential, as well as the potential with each squat of an acute injury.

So what about non-weightlifters? The short answer is that the shallower the squat, the less relevant the toe position is. You can do a quarter squat with your toes turned in without hurting yourself, although this isn't exactly a great idea. An athlete who is squatting only to horizontal or barely breaking horizontal, particularly with the hips-back, limited-knee flexion posture typically used with such squatting, will usually be able to do this with the toes forward because the flexion of the knees is minimal and consequently, the rotation never reaches the degree it would with complete knee flexion. If you insist on squatting with the toes forward, I would recommend keeping the depth limited.

Consider a powerlifting squat (or an archetypal one at least)—the feet are extremely wide, the toes possibly turned out less than many weightlifters', and the depth to horizontal thighs at the greatest. The potential for a knee to drop inward abruptly and injuriously is a real possibility in such a stance because the feet are far outside the knees, meaning the joint is not directly supported by the lower leg. Further, with the toes and knees pointed straight forward, think of the lateral force on the knee (imagine what you would feel in your knees if doing the side splits with your feet elevated and toes straight forward). If you're not very actively pushing out and engaging the lateral hip musculature, you're in trouble. This wide stance and limited outward rotation of the feet also binds up the hip capsule and makes it easier to support the bottom position of the squat. Try a squat with an extremely wide stance and you'll feel what I mean—you'll find that you're forced to stop around parallel because your hips bottom out.

I don't teach a powerlifting squat for a number of reasons not requiring discussion here. My lifters squat with their feet under their thighs. Remember our discussion about aligning the feet and the thigh to ensure proper hinging of the knee—this only works if the feet are under the legs. If they're outside or inside the leg significantly, even with the foot parallel with the thigh, the knee will be forced to rotate. I actually like my lifters' stance to be very slightly outside directly under the legs—this allows the hips to sit slightly between the thighs to help absorb the force at the bottom of the squat somewhat rather than a more abrupt, jarring stop at the bottom as occurs if the thigh and lower leg are perfectly stacked. But this is an extremely minor deviation and creates insignificant rotation at the knee.

Without getting entangled in the interminable weightlifters vs. powerlifters argument, let's consider the weights squatted by each, the positions of those squats and the gear involved. The world record powerlifting squat is over 1000 lbs (more or less depending on the federation). This is fully geared and to approximately parallel depth with a wide stance. Now consider some squats done by weightlifters. One that comes to mind was done by Pat Mendes—an 800-lb squat to full depth with nothing other than neoprene knee sleeves. For those who will argue that it was just bouncing his ass off his calves, how about Mikael Koklyaev squatting 794 lbs relatively slowly with a weightlifting singlet, belt and neoprene knee sleeves—and some impressive depth to boot. The point is simple: even though the absolute weights squatted by weightlifters are lower than the top weights lifted by fully geared powerlifters, weightlifters' knees, hips and ankles are moving through much greater ranges of motion with nearly as much weight and with virtually no supportive gear, and as a consequence, it seems reasonable to state that no other athletes are putting those joints through as much work in the squat. Where are their feet? Nearly invariably pointed out.

In fact, let's not even limit ourselves to weightlifters or deep squats. Take a look at Chuck Vogelphol squatting 1175 or Mike Miller squatting 1220. Feet? Pointed out.

The knees going valgus during a squat has a couple possible causes. One is a squat stance wider than flexibility or anatomy can support—that is, the feet are outside the knees and the knees simply cannot be pushed out far enough to remain over the feet. Another is ankle inflexibility; this will also be accompanied by a wider than desirable stance along with excessive external rotation. In both of these cases, the valgus knee movement will occur during both the eccentric and concentric portions of the squat.

More common is valgus knee movement during only the recovery from the bottom of the squat. If the leg position is correct on the way down, flexibility and stance can't be the problem; in this case, the issue is related to strength and activation of the lateral hip musculature. The athlete is either weak here or for some reason is not properly engaging the muscles necessary to maintain proper positioning and movement. If the athlete is strong and properly engages, there is no need for a particularly high degree of focus on preventing valgus knees; no more focus on this is required than on extending the knees to stand from a squat if the movement is learned and practiced correctly and weaknesses are addressed.

Finally, if the stance is of proper width, valgus knee movement, while not ideal and certainly offering a potential for strain in various locations, is by no means any particularly great opportunity for serious acute injury. The knees are still supported to a large degree by the lower leg vertically—they're not unsupported and buckling in as they would with a squat stance too wide.

Spend some time on youtube watching the elite level weightlifters. You'll notice the overwhelming majority squat with the toes out. Yet ACL tears and strains and other serious acute knee injuries are extremely uncommon among weightlifters, despite the ballistic nature of the majority of their squats.

In short, squatting with the toes out to a correct degree (i.e. not excessive rotation to accommodate ankle inflexibility) and with a proper stance width will not set an athlete up for sudden valgus knee failure, and will in fact help keep the joints moving through their intended planes of motion safely.

Jumping, Landing and Field Play

My knowledge and interest does not extend very far into athletic endeavors outside of competitive weightlifting; however, there are a few points I want to address with regard to this part of the argument.

If we agree that jumping and landing and similar sport-specific actions are best performed with the toes forward, this does not mean we have to agree that the toes-forward position is how we should be squatting. I won't argue with this notion, because not only is this not an area in which I have extensive knowledge, I also have no objection to it.

But gym training does not and cannot perfectly mimic play on the field. If we had to perform exactly in the gym as we did on the field, we could do virtually nothing in the gym. Strength training and the like is intended to develop basic athletic qualities, not finer sport-specific motor patterns—the latter are learned, developed and practiced with sport-specific training on the field. If we're going to say that because we want our football players defaulting to a toes-forward stance, we're going to have them squat this way, that same rationale would need to be applied across the board, which would mean, for example, that we would need them to squat on the balls of their feet rather than with more pressure on their heels because no one sprints or cuts or jumps flat-footed.

To compare the squat to sprinting, jumping and landing is somewhat problematic because of both depth and stance. While landing from a jump may be done in a squat-width stance, both sprinting and jumping will nearly always be performed with a narrower stance. Further, these athletes are not absorbing the force of landing from a jump by squatting—knee and hip flexion is of a limited range of motion. Likewise, neither the support nor the drive of a sprint involves anywhere near the degree of knee and hip flexion seen in a squat. And finally, jumping is not performed from a deep squat position.

Additionally, most of these actions involve primarily single-leg support and drive—the positions of a unilateral leg movement are not identical to a bilateral one. For example, even though I teach my lifters to squat with the toes out, they don't do single-leg work, such as lunging (or splitting in the jerk) with the toes out—but these are different activities that require and allow different positioning. The key to stable unilateral movement and support is strength and control at the hip and ankle—learning to engage the muscles that keep the leg where we want it and making them strong. Interestingly enough, the kind of lateral hip engagement and strength that prevents the knee from going valgus in a single leg support is very similar if not the same used to keep the knees out over externally rotated feet during a bilateral squat.

As far as motor learning goes, consider repetition volume. How many times in a given period is an athlete squatting with the toes out, and how many times in that same period (or over a career) is that athlete jumping, landing or planting a foot and driving in a sprint with the toes oriented as they should be? The volume of the latter eclipses the former by orders of magnitude, and as a consequence, there should be no concern about the motor patterns being altered undesirably.

Athletes need to be taught and practice proper jumping, landing, cutting and footwork mechanics in their sport-specific training, not in the weight room.

Training for Success

The primary goal for any coach or trainer is to prevent your athletes from getting injured. Injured athletes can't play or train. This should always be kept in mind when deciding how to train an athlete. However, there's a difference between training in a manner that prevents injury and one that plans for failure. I prefer the former. In other words, train wisely and safely for success rather than modifying your training to prepare you for impending doom.

Squat in the way you believe and demonstrate to be the safest and most effective for you, and teach your athletes to do the same.

CATALYST ATHLETICS: OUR WARM-UP IS A WARM-UP

Somewhere along the line, warming up became remarkably complicated. And for some, the line between warming up and training has faded to the point that I find myself compelled to say things like the title of this article.

Whenever you start getting confused about what to do, a reliable course of action is to ask yourself a simple question: Why? What is the purpose of this? What am I trying to accomplish? If you can answer those questions, chances are you'll be able to work it all out just fine. If you can't answer those questions satisfactorily, don't be afraid to seek out the advice of someone more experienced in that particular area.

When it comes to warming up, what are we trying to accomplish? The name itself is a bit of a hint, but increasing body temperature is just one element. It might be easier if we rename the *warm-up* to *training preparation*. Now if we ask what we're trying to accomplish, it should be obvious: we're preparing our bodies for the training to follow.

I've seen more times than I can even believe warm-ups that read exactly like workouts—and not easy ones. The first thing I think to myself when I see these warm-ups is that I would have to warm-up to do them. This is a pretty good tip-off that your warm-up may not be serving its purpose. Ring dips, box jumps, burpees and the like are not elements of a warm-up. There will be times when you insert non-warm-up exercises before the primary workout, but these come after an adequate warm-up; they're not part of it. These are usually remedial exercises to address an athlete's or client's weaknesses or activation exercises to help correct inactive musculature in a manner that carries over into the subsequent training (an example would be glute medius activation drills).

The title of this post is a modification of a popular line that demonstrates a lack of understanding of the purpose of a warm-up (which would garner more sympathy from me if it weren't demonstrative of such an elitist attitude), as well as suggests that some people are more concerned with creating the appearance of athletic ability than actually developing it.

Having recently hired two new trainers at Catalyst, I'm having to go over a lot of the fundamentals again to ensure that everyone's on the same page. One of the things I find myself reiterating regularly is that the number one priority in this gym is not hurting people. As much as I feel like this should be so obvious it shouldn't need to be even said out loud, it can be overlooked easily when overwhelmed by the excitement and novelty of certain aspects of training, and often a big part of a trainer's job is protecting clients from themselves.

That being said, I recognize and accept that some injuries and pain are inevitable with any physical activity, particularly among groups of people who have the shared tendency to push themselves. However, I see this not as an excuse to ignore it, but as a reason to do everything we possibly can to minimize the occurrence and severity of injuries. Much of this is accomplished through programming choices and client entry protocols, but the warm-up plays a significant role.

So what should a warm-up actually look like? Here are some guidelines to help you develop what I would consider an effective training preparation protocol.

Monostructural Work

This is some repetitive activity like rowing, jogging or jumping rope. I don't believe this to always be necessary. Its purpose is to get some initial body temperature increase and systemic loosening in unusually cold temperatures or for individuals who have been immobile for a long period of time prior to training. This should be low intensity and for about 2-5 minutes depending on need. We usually start our class warm-ups with one of these or some basic agility ladder drills since most of our clientele work sedentary office jobs. This is definitely important for our early morning classes—usually these clients have literally just rolled out of bed. Agility ladder work is a lot more interesting than jogging or rowing and our clients love it.

Foam Rolling

Possibly the most significant change to my basic warm-up routine has been the addition of pre-training foam rolling. When I was first introduced to the practice, I relegated it to the post-workout period along with stretching. This of course is helpful and certainly worth doing, but rolling before training can make a tremendous impact on movement by allowing muscle and fascia to glide more smoothly. Hitting problem spots a little more aggressively is fine, but generally I suggest pre-training foam rolling be fairly light, smooth and quick rather than slow and painful; the latter I find best saved for after training (this is somewhat analogous to using dynamic stretching pre-workout and static stretching post-workout). I like to hit the upper back to mobilize the thoracic spine, then smooth out the scapular musculature and lat/teres/etc. attachments under the arms. From there glutes, hamstrings/adductors; then VMO/adductors, quads from front to lateral aspects, ITB/TFL, and finally calves if needed. Generally about 10 passes on each area is adequate.

Dynamic Warm-up

This is where we get into the kicks and twirlies. My goal with this portion of a warm-up is two basic things: make sure I address all the movements or joints necessary, and try to get in enough variation day to day that people stay engaged and perform it properly rather than turn into drooling robots who aren't accomplishing what I expect them to.

I posted a video of many of the drills I use frequently on the site a couple years ago. This is a pretty extensive warm-up series and typically I wouldn't actually use all of these in a single warm-up. I think of this stuff in sets of drills that each address a certain movement or area of the body and then I try to alternate exercises each warm-up while still having 1-3 from each set. This is how we get some variety without neglecting anything.

These drills can also be varied to prepare people specifically for the subsequent workout. That is, emphasis can be placed on movements and areas of the body that will be important for the training. An example would be doing more wrist, elbow, shoulder and upper back work for a workout that has a significant overhead component.

I conceptualize these sets or areas of the body somewhat nebulously, but if I had to write them down it would look something like this:

-Wrists
-Elbows
-Shoulders/Upper back
-Spine/trunk
-Hip flexors/quads
-Hip extensors/adductors
-Knees
-Ankles/calves

There is a range of specificity there both by necessity and for the sake of practicality. Following are some ideas of how I address each area. You'll notice that many of the drills don't fit neatly into one category and often address multiple areas—this is just the nature of athletic movement and is only a problem when trying to write something like this. In fact, it ends up being convenient because you're often able to get more accomplished with fewer drills.

Wrists

My default drill here is wrist circles with the hands clasped together. This is quick and simple and usually about as much as the typical person needs. If a client has particularly tight wrists and/or will be doing activity that demands a lot from the wrists, stretches can be done with the hands on the floor or against a wall for flexion and extension or with one hand used to stretch the other. Drills with PVC pipes and similar can also be thrown in occasionally. Also, if you're doing some floor-based work later, e.g. inchworms, you'll be getting some of this stretching along with that.

Elbows

Elbows go overlooked much of the time until they start hurting, at which point it's usually too late to fix them quickly. A few seconds of mobility work will help keep the elbows moving smoothly. Basic elbow circles are usually enough, although I have my clients rotate the hands as they do them to get a little more movement of the radius and ulna. Make sure you go both directions and extend the elbow completely each time.

You can get a bit more involved and throw in things like drill bits or rotations with a PVC pipe. For the latter, hold a PVC pipe horizontally in front of you with your left hand gripping the left end of the pipe with a supinated grip and your right hand grasping the middle of the pipe lightly (doesn't really matter if it's palm up or down, but up is easier). Keeping the right hand as an anchor in about the same place, let the pipe slide through it freely as needed while you pronate your left hand, still gripping the pipe, and extend your left elbow. Move back and forth between supination and pronation, fully extending your elbow each time.

Shoulders/Upper Back

Foam rolling the thoracic spine is the ideal way to start your shoulder warm-up. Many times people are so focused on shoulder mobility that they overlook the fact that their upper backs are hunched and tight, placing excessive demand on the shoulders to take up the slack. Mobilize the upper back, and suddenly your shoulders will feel a lot more flexible.

The basic arm circle forward and backward is the standard. Make sure you're moving the shoulder blades in concert with the arms as you do these and keeping your upper back extended. People get remarkably lazy with these and end up looking like hunchbacks running a giant egg beater in front of themselves. Over and backs (swing the arms up over your shoulders and chop your upper back, then swing the arms back down behind you) and bear hug swings (swing your arms out to the sides, then back across your body like you're hugging yourself) are also quick and easy.

If the following workout is shoulder intensive or the shoulders are a focal point, some more in-depth work can be added. Dislocates and presses behind the neck with a PVC pipe are quick and effective (make sure you're retracting your shoulder blades with the presses). Pipe rolls are a good way to finish after some dislocates. With the same grip, swing one arm up and around your head and follow with the other arm; make sure you go in both directions.

Band pull-downs and chest expanders are good as well. For the pull downs, grip the ends of a light elastic band and hold it overhead like you would a bar for an overhead squat. Keeping the shoulder blades retracted tightly, pull the hands down to the sides until they're below your shoulders. The band should slide lightly down your back—this isn't a dislocate; the hands move straight down and back up. For chest expanders, use the same grip but start with the arms in front of you. Squeeze the shoulder blades back and pull the band apart as you bring your arms backward and let the band stretch across your chest.

Finally, a stretch we call the pat down: get near a wall and put the hands against it overhead like you're getting searched by an arresting officer. Keeping the abs tight to prevent hyperextension of the back, push your chest down and back from the wall to open the shoulders. Instead of just pushing, thinking of pulling down away from the hands as well.

Spine/Trunk

Standing trunk rotations are sufficient to loosen up spinal rotation and hit the hips a bit, and they're quick and nearly impossible to screw up too bad. Allow your back foot to pivot as you rotate away from it. You can do some rotation on the floor with iron crosses, which can be a bit more of a stretch, but doesn't have the same dynamic element; it will, however, work on the ITB and lateral hip. Lying on your back with your arms to the sides and legs straight, lift one straight leg up and then bring it across your body to try to touch it to your opposite hand. Bring it back to the midline and down and switch legs.

While I like the standing rotations a bit more than iron crosses, they can't do what the scorpion can do for the hip flexors. Lying on your stomach with the arms out to the sides, bend one leg and bring the foot to the opposite hand. Activate the glutes as you do this to keep the lower back from hyperextending and to help relax the hip flexors and allow them to stretch.

Hip Flexors/Quads

Leg swings forward and backward are very basic but effective. The back swing will loosen up the quads and hip flexors if done properly: keep the knee close to the other leg and try to close the knee entirely while getting the knee behind the hip.

Lunge variations are excellent for opening up the hips and I like having some kind of lunge used daily not only for this reason but also because of the glute activation and hip stability elements. Basic walking lunges are the simplest, but to this I'll usually add either a rotation of the trunk or lateral trunk flexion toward the lead leg at the bottom of the lunge to further stretch the hip flexors.

Hip circles can be thrown in as well. The glutes should be kept tight as the hips move forward to stretch the hip flexors.

Hip Extensors/Adductors

The bow and bend is again the most basic here but also effective. Bend at the hips with the knees slightly unlocked and reach to the floor, then return to the top and use the glutes to push the hips forward as you lean back. The back can round as you reach down, but don't let it complete the whole movement—make sure the hips are hinging so you're stretching the hamstrings. This will hit the hip flexors quite well also as long as you get the hips through with tight glutes.

The spiderman lunge is one of my top choices for opening up the hips. Take a long lunge step and put the hands on the floor, then try to push your hips and chest toward the floor as far as possible. Stay low as you advance with the next leg. The lead shin should be about vertical—don't get your body way ahead of your front foot. This should feel like someone is trying to rip your leg out of your hip, but in a non-violent and helpful way.

Groiners are like mountain climbers that reach the feet up to the hands and put you in the spiderman lunge position. The idea is to switch legs rhythmically, but to sink in deep each time to stretch out the hip capsule and adductors.

Knees to chest is a good starting movement that doesn't cause much strain. I like doing these walking and extending the ankle of the support leg as you squeeze the other knee to your chest. Make sure the support side glutes are active and your hips remain squared off—don't let the lifted leg side drop.

Lunge variations will do some stretching of the lead leg hamstrings, adductors and glutes. The forward and backward leg swings mentioned above will hit the hamstrings on the forward swing. Lock in the pelvis as you swing—letting the hips rock back simply allows the lower back to flex rather than keeping the swing to the hip joint. Side leg swings will hit the adductors on the outward swing and some lateral hip, TFL and ITB on the inward swing. Lean forward slightly to lean against a wall or pole and swing one leg across yourself and then back out to the side. Let the toe point up at each side.

Inchworms are another good early drill because they're slow and controlled. Place the hands on the floor in front of the feet with straight knees and walk them out slowly. When you reach a push-up position, drop the hips to the floor, engage the glutes, and lift your chest to stretch your hip flexors. Then walk the feet (keeping the legs straight) back up to your hands.

The Kossack is one of those exercises that I love but seem to forget too much of the time. Get into a squat and throw one leg straight out to the side with the heel on the floor and your toes pointed up. Keeping your feet on the floor, shift into a squat on the straight leg side and straighten the formerly bent leg. Keep your hands on the floor in front of you and support yourself as much as you need to make it from side to side without tearing your groin. Eventually you should be able to do this with no arm support and keeping your hips low as you transition from side to side.

Finally, there's the Russian Baby Maker. I doubt I'm the first one to ever do this stretch, but I am the one who gave it that name. And no, I'm not going to explain why—it's an inside joke that dates back to my college years; you'll just have to trust me that it's funny. Put your feet a little wider than your normal squat stance and toes a little more forward than you would normally squat with. With your hands holding the tops of your feet, wedge your elbows between your thighs—get them back as deep into your groin as you can manage. While pushing the elbows out into your thighs, slowly drop your hips toward a squat position. Don't worry about keeping your back arched. This is not the same as pushing the knees out in a squat position—here we're trying to spread the proximal ends of the femurs apart rather than the distal ends. In other words, spread the hips, not the knees. You can hold this bottom position for a while, or you can periodically move the hips up slightly and re-settle.

Knees

The knees should get pretty warm with the above drills, but focus work can be done if desired. Simple squats are a good place to start. To these, you can add some knee rotations in the bottom position, which will also help the hips and ankles. In the bottom of the squat, put the hands on the knees and move the hips up and down slightly as you push the knees in small circles each direction.

You can also do knee rotations in a number of ways from a standing position. The basic one is with the feet close together and straight forward, place the hands on slightly bent knees and move both knees together in a circle. You can also move the feet out and move the knees in the same direction, or in opposite directions.

Ankles/Calves

The above knee circles in the bottom of the squat is a good ankle warm-up and a number of different movements can be performed from this bottom position, such as shifting side to side. A more aggressive stretch can be performed by leaning both forearms on one knee to push the ankle closed.

Ankle circles in the standing position with the toe on the floor are quick and simple, and you can also add some heel-toe walking to other warm-up drills to sneak in some ankle work.

Putting it Together

This isn't an exhaustive list—there are other exercises that can be used to address each of these areas. However, this is more than enough to keep you busy and getting enough variety to not drive yourself or your clients nuts. A single warm-up won't use all of these drills by any means. We get a group warm-up done here in 12-15 minutes at a steady but not rushing pace. An example series might look like:

Wrist circles – 10 each direction
Elbow circles – 10 each direction
Arm circles – 10 each direction
Bow & bend – 10
1-legged RDL + leg swings – 10 each leg
Spiderman lunge – 10 each leg
Scorpion – 10 each side
Russian Baby Makers – 30 sec hold
PVC dislocates – 10
PVC overhead squats - 10

Static Stretching

Select static stretching can be placed here to address specific problem areas that need aggressive stretching.

Corrective Drills

This would now be the time to perform any remedial work you want to place before the workout. The individual is warm and the muscles and joints prepared to perform exercises safely and effectively. Examples would be glute activation drills like bridges, clamshells and X-band walks or shoulder prep/pre-hab work like band external and internal rotations, abduction, etc., or stability exercises like Turkish get-ups. These are drills that will either help the athlete or client perform safely or properly in training, or are elements deemed important enough to warrant the focus and energy only available at the beginning of the training session.

Try It

I know a few people who never warm-up, and a few of them will even tell you that warming up is unnecessary. Interestingly enough, all of these folks have chronic pain and histories of injury. Don't make up silly excuses and analogies because you don't feel like spending a few more minutes getting reading. You're not a wild animal being chased without warning in the jungle—you're an athlete getting ready to train in the gym.

PLANDOMIZATION

Periodization has become a bad word in CrossFit Land. My optimistic view on this phenomenon is that it's due simply to widespread misunderstanding of what exactly periodization is, how variable its implementation can be, and not only its value when used correctly, but its necessity in some form for anyone but the complete beginner. The cynic in me, on the other hand, believes this vehement aversion to periodization of any nature is more a product of frequent bad-mouthing by individuals in positions of authority who fail to grasp the fundamentals and are much more willing to disparage periodization and its proponents and claim a degree of authority so extravagant it exceeds the intellectual capacity of the totality of the world's coaches and athletes, rather than admit a lack of understanding and spend some time learning from others.

Having said this, I feel a need to clarify that I do believe much periodization is constructed poorly and falls short of its intended goals. This, however, demonstrates an individual's ineptitude or inexperience, not a fundamental flaw in the concept itself.

Part of the problem is likely due to the association of specific models with periodization itself; that is, too many people believe periodization to be a particular structure, likely one they've seen in some internet article (or one of those silly digital journals).

Periodization is simply planning. It's creating a structure to guide one's training during a given period of time. It doesn't necessarily mean a progression from higher volume and lower intensity to lower volume and higher intensity, although this basic trend does have a fair degree of utility. In another sense, periodization is the segmentation of training into blocks of time that allow some degree of emphasis on certain traits over others.

Ends & Means

Let me go ahead and distill this entire article to its essence: *If you have no plan with regard to your training, you're an idiot.* Abrasive, I know, but this point needs to sink in.

The idea that you can make maximal progress without a plan in any pursuit, whether it's athletics, business, or space travel, is absurd. Can you make progress without a plan? Sure. You can pretty much guarantee some degree of improvement over a long enough period of time with consistent hard work. But being satisfied with minimal progress when greater progress is entirely achievable is just stupid.

Does this mean everyone needs to know exactly what they'll be doing every day for the next twelve months? Of course not. Planning comes in many different forms and degrees of precision, and those characteristics will vary according to individual needs.

We can plan everything from a single workout, to a short series of workouts in a week, to an entire year of training. How detailed each of these plans is will change according to individual need, but planning on all of these levels should exist in some manner. Without it, we're just crossing our fingers.

Generalization Specifically

CrossFit is a somewhat nebulous program involving "constantly varied, if not randomized, functional movement performed at high intensity." This notion of randomness has become an eclipsing focus of many CrossFit athletes and trainers. Quite possibly this is because approaching training randomly effectively masks a lack of programming ability and gives one a false sense of programming expertise. Anyone can throw a list of exercises and numbers on a whiteboard; far fewer can create workouts that, over a given period of time, ensure an athlete accomplishes his or her goals.

An entirely random approach to training, in my humble, lowly, uneducated opinion, is a mistake. *Being prepared for any random task is not the same thing as preparing randomly for any task.* The importance of this point cannot be overstated.

Being prepared for anything means balancing and improving equally, on average over time, the range of athletic traits. The list created by Jim Cawley of Dynamax is a nice guide: Strength, power, speed, endurance, stamina, flexibility, balance, coordination, agility and accuracy.

This balancing of traits is done by improving one's weaknesses without sacrificing one's strengths unnecessarily until every trait is within a reasonable range of equality, at which time elements can be trained in a more balanced fashion (although emphasis of certain elements during certain times will continue to allow greater progress even in a reasonably balanced athlete). How does one improve one's lacking elements of fitness? By emphasizing those elements in training for given periods of time—not necessarily continuously—until they're no longer weaknesses. Sound like anything we've talked about thus far?

People & Places

We have a few basic kinds of people to consider with regard to all this planning nonsense. First are individuals who must be as balanced as possible—that is, prepared for any contingency—at all times. This includes military personnel, law enforcement officers, firefighters, EMS personnel and the like whose lives and careers depend on being physically capable of managing extreme physical demands without prior notice. A cop doesn't have the luxury, for example, of training for a particularly brutal arrest and control situation on a given date.

Competitive athletes, on the other hand, do have competition schedules and know when and where they'll need their particular set of physical traits. Occasionally athletes like fighters will take on last-minute events other than ones for which they've been preparing, but this is comparatively uncommon, and for these athletes, whether or not to take a fight is ultimately a choice, not a requirement.

Finally we have the vast majority of the exercising population—individuals who seek fitness for its own sake, for health, for improvement of their chosen recreational activities, and even for the enjoyment of training itself. These individuals have no schedule at all, and no need to be prepared in perfect balance at any given moment (an exception might be an individual planning to do something like hike up a big mountain during a family vacation).

The optimist in me believes it should be strikingly obvious that the training needs of these three groups are not the same; the cynic knows that too many of each group have been convinced that they should all be preparing the same way.

Everyone from each of these groups has strengths and weaknesses. Those weaknesses need to be addressed if that individual is to achieve the level of fitness being sought. Again, these things are addressed by emphasizing particular elements—whether specific exercises or entire modalities—in order to bring them up to speed with the remainder of an individual's abilities.

This need to emphasize certain elements doesn't change among individuals, irrespective of career, sport, or hairstyle; what changes is the degree to which one can emphasize a given element over others. In other words, the less the demand for constant readiness, the more we can temporarily and slightly compromise certain abilities for the sake of improving those needing the most improvement.

Compromise

So why should we compromise any element of fitness at anytime? Because in order to genuinely emphasize one element, we need to create slack elsewhere. There is a very real limit to how much the human body can handle simultaneously, and attempting to perform at 100% across the board at all times is a guaranteed recipe for stagnation if not utter disaster.

Interestingly enough, this notion is often dismissed because emphasis and compromise are mistakenly interpreted as specialization and sacrifice. Again, it's critical to understand that it's entirely possible to adjust the degree of emphasis and compromise to be appropriate for any individual in any case.

The fact is that emphasis means greater progress. This cannot be denied without delusion. We can demonstrate this fact by looking to athletic specialists. The strongest athletes in the world, for example, are those who train exclusively for strength and forsake all other elements of fitness that fail to contribute to being stronger in an athlete's event(s). This fact is known to anyone who considers it for a moment, but is often forgotten when entering into passionate discussions regarding fitness.

This rule of emphasis producing greater results can be applied even when fitness is our goal—again, we just modulate the degree of emphasis to better preserve the de-emphasized elements.

An example of this are Michael Rutherford's *Max Effort Black Box* program, which seeks to maintain a rather high level of fitness while emphasizing strength development, and has been very successful with accomplishing this goal. It doesn't sacrifice fitness, and, arguably, actually improves it by increasing the individual's strength, which appears overwhelmingly to be the trait most lacking in CrossFitters. The athlete's performance on longer-duration metabolic workouts may suffer somewhat, but ultimately, such workouts are less builders of fitness than tests of it, and to a large degree, tests of mental fortitude more than physical ability.

The degree of emphasis in a program is commensurate to the degree of comprise. In other words, with more compromise, we can achieve greater improvement in the trait being emphasized (this is not to say that we necessarily need to emphasize/compromise to a great degree in all cases). This rule is important to keep in mind when creating programs to ensure one doesn't mistakenly expect to be able to emphasize to an extent beyond what is allowed by the associated compromise.

Everybody's Doing It

The funny thing (maybe not funny—more exasperating, I suppose) is that nearly every CrossFitter does in fact plan and emphasize certain elements to some extent, knowingly or not (the only ones who don't are the same folks who flail around helplessly in the rest of their lives as well).

I can't do a muscle-up yet and I feel like a tool! I'm going to drop in more ring dips and false-grip ring pull-ups so I can get one. That sounds suspiciously like emphasis and planning.

So it's being done already—the problem is that it's typically not being done well (it's hard to do something well when you either don't know you're doing it or refuse to admit you're doing it). If more people would acknowledge the need to focus on improving their weaknesses, and learn better ways of training to specifically improve them, we'd find not more specialized athletes, but more balanced CrossFitters.

I am a Specialist. At Everything.

Planning is really not that complicated: Determine a goal and decide on a method of achieving it. The key with goal-setting is being reasonable: don't be the guy who makes a goal of adding 50 kg to his back squat in four weeks. It's far more productive to continually make more modest goals, and to continually achieve them on a more frequent basis. This regular accomplishment of goals also keeps the athlete motivated and training hard and consistently, rather than frustrated and training half-heartedly and sporadically.

The generalist will need to have more conservative long-term goals than the specialist, but often short-term goals for generalists can be more ambitious than their specialist counterparts' because those specialists will be far more advanced in their development. In any case, goals need to be limited in number during any given period—the classic rookie mistake is trying to do everything at the same time to the same degree (Sound like anyone you know?).

This is where creating periods of time to focus on different goals comes into play. If we have a CrossFitter who wants to snatch bodyweight, but also wants to be able to add three more rounds to his Cindy, we have two goals that are not remarkably complementary. This athlete is going to get a lot more accomplished if he or she spends some time improving his or her snatch technique and snatch-related strength while preserving metabolic conditioning as well as possible, and then spending some time improving Cindy-specific stamina while preserving his or her new-found snatching ability, than trying to do both together.

This reality is often dismissed with anecdotes of CrossFitters who added 7,000 lbs to their deadlifts while losing 350 lbs of pure fat and dropping 5 minutes off their Fran times—all while simply following the crossfit.com WOD. This argument, of course, fails to consider the remarkable capacity for adaption of untrained or deconditioned individuals, and the comparatively limited capacity of individuals with many years of smart training under their belts. If an individual is untrained enough, I can improve his deadlift with nothing more than vigorous nose-picking. The point is, what works for beginners (which is anything at all) doesn't work for more advanced athletes. The more advanced an athlete is, the closer he or she is to his ultimate capacity, and the more necessary legitimate planning becomes. Again, for demonstration of this, look to athletic specialists.

Plandomization

Part of CrossFit's effectiveness is the constant variation of the metabolic workouts in terms of exercises, reps, rounds, etc. (as an aside, its biggest weakness is the constant variation and random implementation of strength work).

So how do we reconcile this notion of constant variation with planning for specific goals? Simple: we plan the fundamental structure of our training—the training that is helping us accomplish our current primary goal—and fill in the spaces with more randomized—but smart—training that takes into consideration our secondary goals.

Most often what this will look like (or should look like, considering the current state of CrossFitters at large) is a structured strength program accompanied by CrossFit-style metabolic workouts. These workouts will be varied continually, but they should not be randomly created. At minimum, these workouts should be constructed in a manner than doesn't interfere with the strength work; ideally, they should be constructed with an effort to work toward accomplishing a secondary goal.

A secondary goal needs to be kept just that—it's easy to get carried away and attempt to achieve too much at once, which nearly always results in failure across the board. Secondary-goal-oriented programming would be the emphasis of exercises or elements that have proven to be weaknesses for the athlete in question within actual CrossFit workouts. This might look like increased frequency of pull-ups in metCons for individuals whose pull-ups are lagging, or an increase in box jump height for an athlete who realizes he or she has been sandbagging with little girl boxes and needs to actually put effort into jumping. It may be spending a few more minutes before and after every workout on flexibility and mobility, or taking a little ego hit and performing dumbbell cleans instead of power cleans in order to shore up bottom-position weakness.

In other words, it doesn't need to involve any kind of extravagant planning—simply being cognizant of minor weaknesses and ensuring such exercises or elements don't continue to be neglected. As those elements improve sufficiently, we move on to the next crop of weaknesses.

This is exactly how I approach the CrossFit programming at Catalyst Athletics. I can tell you exactly what strength work our CrossFitters will be doing six Tuesdays from now, but I can't tell you what metCon they'll be doing that day yet. I plan seven-week strength cycles, but I plan each week's metCons the week prior. When creating these metCons, I consider the strength workout on the same day and the rest of the week, the other metCons that week, and the metCons from prior weeks, along with the weaknesses and strengths I see in our clients; additionally, I modulate volume and intensity appropriately and make sure that all types of movement are adequately represented. Based on my observation of the clients, I have goals for them, both short- and long-term, and I create workouts and workout series to accomplish these goals. In other words, while the metCons are constantly varied, they're by no means random or thoughtless.

Work on It

This article is more of an attempt to motivate smarter programming by CrossFit athletes and trainers than to provide actual guidance for such programming. Guidance of that nature requires far more information than can be contained in an article like this—it requires active pursuit of pertinent information, experimentation, and discussion with other professionals.

If you believe you know all there is to know about programming, you haven't done your homework. There is always more information out there, and there will always be someone who knows something you don't. Learn to be unsatisfied with your current abilities.

ELIMINATING THE STOPWATCH

One of the defining characteristics of CrossFit training is the use of a stopwatch or clock to time workouts. This practice is often regarded as being integral to the effectiveness of the training by turning each workout into a competition and making training "measurable". I've used this approach in the past; prior to my introduction to CrossFit, I never used it with myself or my clients; and as of about a year ago, we no longer time workouts at Catalyst Athletics—even ones that taste a bit like CrossFit.

The stopwatch on workouts has bothered me for quite some time, but I ignored it for a couple years, working around the related problems in every possible way except the most obvious and sensible—removing the stopwatch.

We now give our clients the option to time their own workouts, but our trainers don't do it. Interestingly enough, very few of our clients time their workouts even with this option available. When we do an actual CrossFit workout (once ever couple months or so, we use one of the few good old diagnostic workouts: Cindy, Diane, Fran, Helen and Jackie), we time it—in that case, a time is actually useful for clients to compare previous performances.

My problems with the stopwatch:

1) The only competition clients have while exercising is themselves, both metaphysically and practically. We can pretend that our clients are competing against each other in some kind of sport, but their times are meaningless unless all of your clients are duplications of the same person with the same abilities using the same weights.

2) I don't care how much you emphasize proper exercise execution—once someone is racing a clock, they will sacrifice movement for speed. If you buy into the CrossFit notion that work capacity / power output trumps all, this doesn't matter. If you disagree with the philosophy, it's a serious problem. I believe that movement and the manner in which it's performed is extremely important—much more so than some nebulous idea of work capacity.

3) Not having an actual clock on your workout doesn't prevent you from pushing the pace. However, not having a clock does help you focus on

what's most important.

4) Times from workouts seem to dominate in terms of importance in clients' minds when instead they should be paying attention to the loads they're using, the accuracy of their movements, the type and magnitude of exertion and just about anything else other than time.

5) If your training is set up to be constantly varied and you never repeat a workout, what utility is a time? There's nothing to compare it to.

Can you train well while timing everything you do? I'm sure it's possible; it's just tough to do, and even tougher to ensure others are doing. My first stage in getting rid of the clock at Catalyst Athletics was removing it from our introductory class series—new clients never had a workout timed until they finished this series and entered the open classes. By that time, we had instilled in them a sense of priorities. If you decide to keep the clock running, I would strongly encourage keeping new clients off the clock during their initial period of training.

TEACHING THE OLYMPIC LIFTS IN THE CROSSFIT SETTING

Sometimes your clients are confused. It's true. Some want to squat to big padded balls instead of just learning where their asses are and squatting like grown-ups all the way to the bottom. Some want to do low-bar back squats. And some aren't very interested in learning the snatch and clean & jerk. Fortunately, as a trainer or coach, it's your responsibility to train your clients according to what they need rather than what they want—if they knew what they needed, they wouldn't be your clients.

This is not to say that as a trainer you get to determine your clients' goals—it means simply that the reason someone is paying you is to determine how best to achieve those goals and to lead them through the process. This often means their doing certain things they may not want to do initially.

When it comes to complex lifts like the snatch and clean & jerk, this lack of interest can make learning a difficult and comparatively unsuccessful endeavor. At least part of the issue is that many in CrossFit—both on the client and trainer levels—don't understand the extent of the lifts' complexity, and consequently fail to put in adequate time and effort to learning both the lifts execution and methods of teaching them. This magnifies the silliness described previously and leads to behavior such as celebrating lift performances like those seen during the snatch event of the last CrossFit Games.

In addition to this, teaching the Olympic lifts in a group setting in which they're not only not the primary focus of training, but in which individuals are typically all at different levels of experience, skill, motivation, strength, flexibility and similar factors, becomes far more complicated and frustrating.

In order to address both basic problems described above, we can create a system of teaching the lifts that accommodates different levels of ability, reduces time dedicated to the lifts within any given training session—which allows a breadth of training as well as minimizes the possible effects of clients' disinterest in the lifts and consequent lack of focus and effort—yet not only remains effective, but is arguably more effective than more focused teaching approaches.

Building the Foundation

The finer details of the teaching system employed by each gym will vary just as

GREG EVERETT

all other details of training with vary among CrossFit gyms. There are numerous possible approaches to teaching the lifts in such a setting, and which is used and most effective will vary depending on factors such as how exactly the group training program is administered and the relative emphases on various training components. For example, a gym with a relatively small and consistent clientele is able to do things differently than one with a large and less consistent clientele. Similarly, a gym that emphasizes strength work will have better options than one that uses the common Jazzercise approach of random and extended metabolic workouts with equally random and infrequent strength work. That's another article altogether, but suffice to say if your gym falls into the latter category, you have some fundamental restructuring to do before really worrying about getting this jiggy with the Olympic lifts specifically.

Get Perspective

The first step in develop such a teaching system is learning to consider training in the long term. The failure to do this is a common problem in CrossFit gyms, resulting in random or arbitrary programming that is unable to address long term progress. Your clients will not be training for only a day or a week—why would you approach their training plan in such a term?

Know What You're Doing

This is a fairly important one. If you don't understand the Olympic lifts and how they should be executed, you have no business teaching them to your clients. A Level 1 certification and some CrossFit Journal videos are not an adequate background. There's nothing wrong with such a background—what's wrong is believing or insisting that it prepares you to teach and coach the lifts. Have the integrity as a professional trainer to recognize this and do your homework. Learn more and get better by working privately with qualified weightlifting coaches and attending seminars. (I know of a decent book that might be helpful too.)

Until that point, bring in an outside coach to work with your clients occasionally in a seminar or occasional class format; if this isn't possible stick with the exercises you know how to teach. Anything else is a disservice to your clients, who are likely paying you handsomely for your presumed expertise. They will respect and appreciate you far more for admitting your lack of expertise in a particular special area, than for teaching them poorly. You don't have to be the greatest weightlifting coach in the world—you do need to have a solid grasp of the fundamentals to avoid teaching your clients so many of the ridiculous things they find out later they have to change.

Have a Plan

This ties in with gaining perspective. Figure out what you're doing before you start doing it. This saves everyone time and frustration, and allows far more effective teaching. Having a plan doesn't necessarily mean that even the most minute details are in print three months prior to starting—it means having a level of detail sufficient to guide you to your intended goals. This plan can be flexible, and must be to some extent considering the setting about which we're talking, but at no time should the approach be arbitrary or based on what you happen to feel like doing at the moment.

Shaping the System

Whatever system is finally established, it must take into account a few key elements:

> Different skill levels among clients in a class
> Regular influx of new clients
> Inconsistent training schedules of clients
> Available time in training sessions for this component
> Attention span of clients
> The role of the lifts in the overall program

Different Skill Levels

Unless a gym brings on new clients in a structured group format like Nicki Violetti's On-Ramp program, and subsequently keeps these clients locked into given class times for the duration of their membership, there is bound to be a broad spectrum of skill and experience among clients in a class (even with such a rigid approach, different clients learn more quickly and perform better than others). With any system for teaching the lifts, we need to be able to accommodate all of these clients, not just teach to a certain level because it's simplest for us. This is easily the most difficult aspect of the process.

The ideal way to address this problem would be to separate clients into different classes based on demonstrated ability. Such stratification is immensely helpful with respect to all aspects of training, but is often very impractical. It means limiting, often greatly, the number of possible classes for each client, while simultaneously increasing the burden of the trainers. There are few gyms that are able to make such a structure work. However, few if any gyms should be unable to separate the absolute beginners from the rest of the clientele—this again can be accomplished by using a system of entry to the program like the On-Ramp classes. This alone makes the task of teaching the lifts far easier and more effective by simply removing the least skilled clients from the equation. They don't factor in until they've achieved a basic level of proficiency with fundamental exercises.

The next best option would be multiple trainers working with the clients in a given class so those clients can be grouped together according to skill level and lead through different training during a single class. While somewhat more practical than separating actual classes, this is still difficult and expensive.

Instead, we need to find a way to have clients function independently enough that a single trainer can run a class without sacrificing the effectiveness of their training or the trainer's ability to provide the necessary instruction. This can really only be accomplished with a genuine plan and structure as discussed previously. In general terms, this means simply determining how much skill variation exists among the clients of a given gym, deciding how many levels of instruction are required to accommodate all of those clients, and then what exactly each skill level will be working on during a given training session. The details of this will be filled out later in the article.

Influx of New Clients

The regular influx of new clients to a CrossFit gym is the source of numerous problems with regard to class structuring and instruction. How this affects the instruction of the Olympic lifts specifically will vary depending on how a gym channels these new clients. A facility that simply jumps new clients into existing classes will have a far more difficult time than one that takes new clients through some sort of introductory class series to establish fundamental exercise proficiency, a base level of work capacity, and a general understanding of how to function as a client within a group training environment. Again, the ideal way of addressing this problem is to use some type of introductory system like an On-Ramp program that separates rank beginners from the rest of the crowd.

Inconsistent Training Schedules

Often one of the most frustrating and limiting aspects of CrossFit style group training is the inconsistent training schedules of the clients. That is, some may come three days each week, and some six; some may come on the same days and times each week, while others show up randomly. This of course makes programming a far more difficult task, and unavoidably reduces the effectiveness of the program for individual clients.

While we can't control clients' attendance, we can prioritize clients and channel our time and efforts accordingly. Our commitment as trainers and coaches should reflect the commitment of our clients—those clients who go out of their way to attend frequently and regularly and train with focus and dedication deserve more attention and effort than those who attend inconsistently and appear to be interested in little more than post-spastic-workout euphoria.

This means programming with your priority clients in mind. This can be done literally—considering the schedules and needs of actual priority clients—or using a theoretical model of your ideal client (as long as it's reasonable). For example, we may program with a consistent 5-day weekly client in mind and simply be flexible for clients who don't fit into this category.

Available Time

How much time in each training session is available for Olympic lift instruction will obviously shape to a large degree what we do. Ideally the instruction and practice of the lifts is taken into consideration when designing the overall structure of the gym's program rather than it being an afterthought. If it is, this will be far less of an issue because adequate time will always be available. If it's not, we will have to work around silliness like medicine ball cleans and sumo deadlift high-pulls in obscene quantities. This just means less time to dedicate to the important things in life like skill and strength.

Client Attention Spans

CrossFitters tend to have comparatively limited attention spans—this characteristic is part of the attraction to a training system that prides itself on constant variation, extremely brief workouts and goals that are by design entirely nonspecific. This needs to be taken into account when designing a system of teaching involved and complex movements, particularly when so many clients will have been convinced that the Olympic lifts are not actually technically complex and can be taught adequately in three minutes with a medicine ball.

Part of solving this problem is educating and re-educating your clients regarding the lifts and their role in their training. If your gym's program, from the beginning of each client's exposure, emphasizes the importance of technical proficiency, strength and Olympic lifts, structured programming, and long term planning, you can expect little if any resistance. If instead your program evolves into this from the Jazzercise type of random metabolic conditioning workouts with infrequent and equally random strength training, clients may have difficulty with the transition simply because they're not accustomed to the new format.

As the trainer, it's your responsibility to stand by your decision. Don't feel obligated to explain why the change is being made unless asked. Sputtering on about training theory to clients who aren't interested simply makes you appear unsure about what you're doing and why you're doing it. It's easy to be confident regarding your programming if you develop it logically; if you're not confident in your gym's program, you have some serious re-evaluation and restructuring to do.

This will in part, along with the role of the lifts discussed next, determine how involved and technical the instruction of the lifts is. That is, shorter attention spans mean more focus on drills to teach the body how to lift and less focus on actual technical education regarding the finer details and reasons why.

Role of the Lifts

A final consideration when developing your training system is what role the Olympic lifts play in the overall training program. That is, how much emphasis is placed on them relative to other lifts and other types of training, and how will they be used—independently as real lifts, within metabolic workouts, or both. Additionally, this will be part of the determination of how technical teaching is. The greater the role the lifts play in the program, the more technical their instruction will need to be in order to improve clients' execution.

The Lifts within the Training Program

All this talk of mixed skill levels and the importance of technical proficiency begs the question: How do we use the Olympic lifts within metabolic conditioning workouts in a group? The easiest answer is not to. The reality is that the overwhelming majority of CrossFit clients will never reach a level of technical proficiency that makes the lifts' use within metabolic workouts a great idea, simply because the proportion of their training time dedicated to the lifts is minimal.

There are better options for conditioning that won't hinder further development of lift technique while still providing a large metabolic dent—arguably more of one, in fact. Additionally, dumbbell, sandbag, and other implement variations of the Olympic lifts can be used to provide most of the metabolic effects desired from the lifts—these lifts require far less instruction and practice to be effective and are distinct enough to not interfere with technique for the barbell lifts. (It should be noted that these exercises do not include the medicine ball clean, because it is hopelessly lame and has no place in anyone's training.)

Within a CrossFit gym with clients who have established reasonable technical proficiency with the barbell Olympic lifts, these lifts can be used within conditioning workouts if desired (although I heartily discourage it). The solution to mixed skill levels within a class is to simply scale the workouts with respect to exercise variation—for example, the top-tier clients may snatch; a middle-tier may 1-arm dumbbell snatch; and a bottom-tier may do jumping dumbbell squats and/or overhead squats. This allows the more advanced athletes to train more effectively, and allows the more novice athletes to train more appropriately without separating them entirely—this helps foster a team atmosphere by keeping everyone performing a similar workout in essence, but doesn't compromise individual clients' training.

Part 2

Before we continue on this particular adventure, I want to provide some clarification on a few items from the first part of the article. It has been pointed out to me that some of my remarks offended certain individuals, and because this was not my intention, I'm going to take a moment to apologize for any offense that was taken, and to provide my rationale for those remarks. While I may make jokes of certain things, my opinions on them are never without reason.

These reasons are not ones pulled from the ether—they are based on the sum of my training experiences, both in and out of CrossFit. My experience with CrossFit itself dates back to some time in early 2004 when I started working with CrossFit coach extraordinaire, Robb Wolf, and shortly thereafter became a partner in CrossFit NorCal, the fourth affiliate. I had been a credentialed trainer for six years prior to this, but very quickly saw CrossFit as not only an amazing training system, but a community that was beginning to attract the kind of coaches and athletes with whom I wanted to interact, learn and improve (stunning how much things have changed since that time). This included people like Robb, Michael Rutherford (CF Kansas City) and Mike Burgener. To this day, these people are some of the greatest contributors to my education as a trainer and athlete, and are good friends—one of the greatest aspects of CrossFit.

Since my start with NorCal, I've had a lot of time to experiment with and evaluate various CrossFit-related protocols with my own clients, as well as to discuss such things with other trainers in and out of the CrossFit community. It is on this collective experience that I base my opinions—not whim, fashion or convention.

The Low-Bar Back Squat

Let's take care of this one first since it's such a popular topic. Most readers of the PM are likely already familiar with my opinion regarding the low-bar back squat, and particularly its use by weightlifters.

Generally I confine my opinion regarding the LBBS to weightlifting, but let me turn over another stone and explain my aversion to it for the generalist. First, if you are a generalist, do it… sometimes. Don't replace the back squat with it completely. I say this not because I like the LBBS for the generalist, but because as a generalist, the more exposure you have to more exercises, the better off you'll be. In my opinion, its use should be infrequent and more as a tool for achieving occasional variety than as a staple exercise. I see it the same way I see the box squat—it has a purpose, it can be legit in the right circumstances, but it's not an exercise on which to build a training foundation.

The reasons for this can be found partly in the aforementioned article, but obviously there's more to it since we're not talking about weightlifters here. In short, the squat is the only potential full knee and hip range of motion strength exercise—the bottom position of the LBBS limits the range of motion of the knee and prevents an opportunity for the quad to open the knee joint in its most mechanically disadvantaged angles. We can combine the LBBS with the front squat, of course, to accommodate this desire for complete knee flexion and greater quad reliance, but two problems arise. First, it's a different lift—in a sense more of a core exercise than a leg and hip exercise. Second, individuals whose only other squat is the LBBS invariably perform the front squat poorly. This is due in part to having trouble reconciling the movement pattern of the LBBS with that of the front squat; the former involving an active backward drive of the hips, and the latter requiring simultaneous knee and hip flexion with as direct of a downward path for the hips as possible. This results in front squats with the hips swinging back on the way up and down, which pulls in more posterior chain and reduces the work for the quads, changing the effect of the exercise (and ultimately limiting loading).

The technical causes of this problem can of course be corrected through coaching and practice, but the strength-related causes are more difficult to correct. For an individual who emphasizes the posterior chain through squatting and pulling exercises, the requisite quad strength will simply not exist to maintain the upright posture and hip path that we're after in the front squat. This leads to the poor performance described above, which simply reinforces the current strength disparity around the knee.

Contributing to this problem is the deadlifting and Olympic lift pulling postures typically employed by generalists who use the low-bar back squat. These pulling postures are also designed to emphasize posterior chain contribution and limit knee involvement.

This prevalence of posterior-chain emphasis strength work fails to balance the quad-dominance it is often claimed to be correcting, and simply swings the pendulum to the other side, creating the kind posterior-chain dominance that prevents desirable front squat and Olympic lift mechanics. This limits an individual's athletic development by retarding progress in the lifts and placing too much emphasis on certain elements, positions and movements. For the generalist, attempting to improve in all respects, this should be quite clearly a problem.

Squatting to Balls

The use of medicine balls as depth gauges for squats is not one I endorse, and one I have admittedly ridiculed—not with intentions of insulting anyone in particular, more to make a point that happens to involve what some find funny. There are times very early in the learning stages for some clients during which achieving adequate depth in a squat is difficult, and during which the client's sense of his or her depth is not accurate. In such cases, one method of encouraging better depth, teaching a sense of position, and better engaging the glutes and hamstrings is to have such clients squat to an object of appropriate height.

This practice is not one I object to, because it can be quite effective. That said, a medicine ball is not, in my opinion, an appropriate object for this. If a client is having difficulty of a degree and nature that necessitates this method of teaching and practice, a ball is not only generally too low of a target, but more importantly, is not a stable and reliable platform to support that client should he or she crash at the bottom. If you have a client who is unstable, weak and in such little control over his or her body that they need to be squatting to a target, the last thing you want is that target being one that allows a fall and actually magnifies the potential for damage.

Medicine balls roll, compress, and otherwise provide an unreliable target; more importantly, their height is not adjustable, and no one can tell me with a straight face that people of all statures and abilities should be squatting to an identical depth. Boxes provide a stable, consistent and reliable target and platform for support if needed, and their height can be easily adjusted appropriately for an individual by stacking plates or similar items on top or underneath.

Finally, if as a trainer you decide to use a box in the early stages of teaching an individual to squat, it should be confined to that stage—it is a temporary tool to achieve a specific set of goals. To continue using anything once an athlete is able to squat to proper depth—especially a ball that rolls, allows an individual to bounce, and is very unlikely the proper height—is a disservice to your clients, who need to eventually develop a reliable sense of position on their own. The concepts of "elite" and "unaware of ass location" cannot describe the same individual. (And of course, as was alluded to in the remarks contained in the first part of this article, actually squatting all the way down makes this much less of an issue—it's pretty difficult to not recognize when your hamstrings are pressed against your calves.)

Sumo Deadlift High-Pull

I lumped this exercise in with medicine ball cleans as "silliness" I ostensibly wouldn't allow with my own clients. This is a minor objection, but my view is simply this: Why not just perform a deadlift high-pull? What advantage does a sumo stance provide for this exercise other than making it easier, and why would we want to make it easier? If, for conditioning, we're interested in moving large loads long distances quickly, why would we shorten the distance we can possibly move the weight, and particularly in a manner that reduces the work of the legs and hips but maintains the work of the shoulders and arms?

I actually use kettlebell deadlift high-pulls in our On-Ramp program, but following those few exposures, it rarely comes up again. Once out of the beginning stages of learning, our clients no longer need such an exercise—they can deadlift, clean, snatch and the like with various implements. I'm not completely averse to ever doing high-pulls, as I do feel they have their place in certain situations, but the reality is that in large and frequent doses, they encourage habits that interfere with clean and snatch technique, which is already difficult enough to teach to generalists. The SDHP is absolutely not an acceptable substitute for the clean, and it should not be considered a part of a teaching progression for the clean. It is strictly a metabolic workout exercise, and, in my opinion, is not one of the better options available.

Level 1 Certifications and the Olympic Lifts

I'm actually not sure if my remarks on this topic were among those not taken well by certain individuals, but in the interest of thoroughness, I'll address it anyway. First, I'm not interested in critiquing the curriculum of CF certifications. It's not my business, and I'm happy to leave the decisions to those who make a living running them—I'm going to assume they have good reason for doing what they do how they do it, and that their guiding intention is creating what they feel are the best fitness trainers possible. My point was actually quite simple, and disagreement with it would absolutely baffle me—the Level 1 certification does not prepare trainers to teach the snatch and clean & jerk, and to insist otherwise is completely irresponsible.

CrossFit trainers who want to become competent in teaching the Olympic lifts need—at the very least—to attend one of Coach Burgener's weightlifting certifications. The reality is that no two-day seminar, even on a single topic with an incredible coach like Burgener, can provide as much instruction, practice and experience as is needed to become genuinely competent in instructing the lifts. It should be considered one part of an ongoing process. In fact, I strongly encourage trainers to attend Burgener's cert more than once if possible—the second time through will be even more enlightening with the experience accumulated since the first. This being said, it should be fairly obvious that a two-day seminar that barely touches on the Olympic lifts certainly cannot create great weightlifting coaches. This just means, as one of our weightlifters, Steve, likes to say, *staying in your lane*—teach what you know, and continue to learn more.

Not being an expert in the Olympic lifts does not make you a bad trainer—posing as an expert to the detriment of your clients does. The experience level of new CrossFit trainers generally parallels that of their clients; that is, trainers will be able to continually improve their experience and abilities at a pace that keeps up with the needs of their clients. It's unnecessary to reach beyond one's scope of experience, then; clients will be better served by instruction and practice of the fundamentals before venturing into more advanced movements.

The Complexity of the Olympic Lifts

Related to the previous was my comment of the general under-recognition by CrossFitters of the technical complexity of the snatch and clean & jerk. This actually can be attributed to a number of sources; let me just say that it's not a surprise when the lifts are given little attention, both within training and in terms of instruction—such a perspective can be expected to develop. Again, trainers are encouraged to spend time with weightlifting coaches and weightlifters—training, watching, talking. Exposure to the weightlifting community directly is the best (and arguably only) way to develop a sincere appreciation for the level of skill required for technical proficiency in the lifts.

This should not be misunderstood as an expectation of generalists to become expert weightlifters—by definition of the term *generalist*, that would be impossible. It is an expectation, however, that generalists place appropriate emphasis on developing snatch and clean & jerk technique. It should be obvious that the elements of an individual's training that require the most skill require the most practice: the Olympic lifts and the handful of basic gymnastics movements are these elements. Once an individual can perform a thruster, how much practice does he or she really need with it? The only necessary exposures to the movement after it's learned are those in which it's used for training purposes. The snatch and clean & jerk, on the other hand, cannot be mastered in a similar manner and timeframe. Weightlifters perform the competition lifts and variations thereof generally 4-6 days each week, sometimes multiple times each day, for years on end, and continue emphasizing technique improvement. There is not a single CrossFitter, present, past or future, who would not benefit from more coaching and practice in the lifts.

At least once I've heard it said that the Olympic lifts don't even compare in complexity to gymnastics movements. I'll be the first to agree, if we're talking about the entire collection of competitive and training movements. Within the realm of CrossFit, however, gymnastics movements are restricted to a handful of extremely basic ones that certainly don't rival the complexity of the snatch and clean & jerk.

The CrossFit Games Snatch Event

This one may have stung a bit for a number of people, and for that I apologize, but my assessment is not one arising from anything but what I feel are reasonable expectations of a community that strives for and claims the status of *elite*. The snatch is a competitive exercise that conforms accordingly to a number of technical rules. These rules are not exclusively for the sake of competition, however—there are elements of execution that are important for the sake of athletic development. Two extremely basic ones are that no part of the body other than the feet can contact the ground, and that the bar must be received and held overhead with fully extended elbows. Both of these were violated repeatedly by many competitors, often dramatically. In fact, it seemed at times, the greater the violation, the more people were impressed.

Having said all this, part of the problem could have been resolved by simply not calling the event a snatch—call it a *ground to overhead anyhow*, and I have no serious complaints. However, if the precision of the exercise is removed, so is much of the point. If the goal is to simply move weight with no concern for how, there are better ways to do it, which move more weight. The only reason I can imagine to hold a snatch event is to distinguish athletes further along in their development to those less experienced—those who have put in the time and effort to develop greater skill than the next athlete. Once you remove the technical requirements, it's simply another strength event—so why not squat, press, etc. instead?

Jazzercise

If you as a gym owner or programmer have no plan, no long-term perspective, no underlying structure and only infrequent and random strength work, you're failing to tap into CrossFit's true potential and are doing your clients a disservice. If this hurts your feelings, quit being satisfied with the easy approach, do your homework, and strive to continue improving the service you provide.

Finally—The Medicine Ball Clean

Of all my potentially offensive remarks, this one may have been the most offensive because of its role in the Level 1 curriculum and its use by many CrossFit gyms. My objection to this, despite the opinions of certain individuals, is actually for very specific reasons.

There are a few relatively minor issues that still manage to chap my ass. One is the head position the athlete is forced to assume with the ball in the "rack" position—tilted way back to make room for the ball. More important is the rack position itself—there is no rack. The ball is supported entirely in the arms, which is understandable to some extent, but the ball is racked with the elbows straight down—not exactly a great habit to be developing for future grown-up cleans. Related to this is the elbow movement of the pull under the ball, which is taught as back and around rather than initiating the pull with the up and out elbow direction that is necessary to pull under a heavy clean. Again, these are comparatively minor problems, but problems nonetheless, and when the ostensible goal is to teach a complex movement as quickly as easily as possible (presumably accurately, as well), it makes little sense to create habits that must be unlearned later.

Next is the instruction to shrug the ball up at the top of the leg and hip extension. Not only should the shrug not be occurring at this point, the manner of teaching encourages hesitation at the top of the extension, which is not a problem when one is cleaning a 20 lb padded ball, but will quite effectively prevent a successful clean with significant weights. The athlete needs to be taught to change directions following leg and hip extension as quickly as possible, and needs to understand that the shrug occurs as he or she is moving down under the implement—it does not elevate the implement. Using an odd-object for an individual's initial exposure to the clean teaches poor body position and stiff arms directed away from the body.

The progression is simply backward. An individual who can clean a barbell can clean anything; an individual who has only cleaned a medicine ball can clean things that look and feel like medicine balls, and only do that in the manner in which one can clean a medicine ball. The transferability is bordering on nonexistent. It makes no sense at all to teach a medicine ball clean when one can in the matter of minutes teach a dumbbell clean, which can be taught and executed in a manner that closely resembles a barbell clean, will not interfere with later learning of the barbell clean, will provide quality training effects, and actually has the potential for some legitimate loading.

Finally, if, as CrossFit trainers and athletes, we're so elite, why can't we even teach or perform a barbell clean correctly?

Part 3

Now that we got all that silliness out of the way, we can get back to talking shop. But first—the last parts of this article received some comments regarding the lifts' use within CrossFit conditioning workouts that warrant response. A sentiment that seems to be shared by a number of CrossFitters (presumably the majority) is that the snatch and clean & jerk are used by CrossFitters for different reasons than by weightlifters (this much is obvious)—namely, as a method of moving large loads long distances in little time for the sake of "increasing work capacity across broad time and modal domains." This, it's argued, means that technical proficiency is simply unnecessary—it doesn't matter how the weight gets from A to B as long as it does so quickly.

I'm not going to lie—this line of reasoning is thoroughly exasperating. A weightlifter's goal is to snatch and clean & jerk as much weight as possible. To this end, he or she continues improving strength, speed and technical proficiency. The more precise a lifter's technique, the more he or she is able to snatch or clean & jerk, because the more effectively his or her strength and speed is applied. This is not a confusing concept—lift technique is designed to allow the athlete to apply maximal force to elevate the bar, get under it, and recover. A lifter can continue getting stronger and faster, but these qualities will never be optimally applicable without equivalently developed technique.

For the CrossFitter—even one who desires only to snatch and clean & jerk some astronomical number of consecutive repetitions—technical proficiency means more weight lifted in less time, as well as a reduction in extraneous effort due to inconsistent positions and movements among reps, or, for example, Sots pressing a failed snatch off the dome. This means more work can be done in a given period of time, whether that period is defined as the time to execute a single lift or a series of them, and consequently "increased work capacity across broad time and modal domains."

If it doesn't matter how the bar gets from A to B (this is the same argument used to support the use of the kipping pull-up, in case you're getting confused— same start and end points, meaning same vertical mass displacement, meaning same approximate amount of work performed, but faster movement, meaning more power), then why would there possibly be any resistance to improving the method of elevating that bar in a manner befitting the stated goals?

Surely it can't be argued that there isn't enough time to work on lift technique—CrossFit workouts take less time than many bowel movements. Quit resisting improvement, develop some perspective, and do a bit of work. And if you're going to argue, at least have the courtesy to come up with some legitimate rationale (actually don't waste your time—it doesn't exist).

Designing the System

Knowing what we now know, we need to create a system of instructing and practicing the Olympic lifts that addresses all of the complications discussed in the first part of the article. As has been mentioned a number of times, the actual system will vary among gyms, so instead of making a rigid prescription, I'm going to simply provide an example that can be used as a template and reshaped to fit various applications.

This example takes into consideration the setup of our own CrossFit program—ours is one that emphasizes strength and technical proficiency. I design a moderate-term strength program (generally 6-8 weeks) that involves 1-2 strength or Olympic lifts per training day prior to conditioning workouts, which are relatively brief and designed largely around the strength program.

We bring in new clients through an On-Ramp program, which means we don't have any absolute beginners to worry about when doing this strength and Olympic lift work. All clients by this point are able to front, back and overhead squat, deadlift, press and push press quite well, with some exception in cases of extreme inflexibility that has not yet been resolved, or particularly poor motor skill. Not once have we had a client complain or ask why we do things the way we do, as this is what we have accustomed them to from day one, and because they continue to make excellent progress.

The following system also takes into account the fact that our clients are adults and treated as such with the according responsibility. For example, our clients bring their own notebooks and record all of their workouts. This means that they know what they've done on any given date, and we don't have to waste everyone's time trying to remember weights, reps, times or guessing when we shouldn't be.

Nuts & Bolts

The first step is determining what drills and exercises we want to use in the instruction and practice process. Anyone involved with CrossFit should be aware of at least one teaching progression—Coach Burgener's. This can be used in the following system, but obviously I'm going to use my own in this example. If the Burgener Warm-up is what you're accustomed to and comfortable with, use it (but please do it correctly—and if you don't do it correctly, please don't post videos of it all over YouTube). It should be fairly clear how to substitute the BWU drills with mine.

It's important to continue with the long term perspective when considering the following process. With this approach, clients won't be performing certain lifts for a while into their training careers, but unless we expect them to train for only a couple months, this shouldn't be a concern. And if they do only train for a couple months, they probably don't deserve your time and effort anyway.

Because by the time our clients are first exposed to the Olympic lifts they have already been taught and have been practicing the back squat, front squat and overhead squat, our basic receiving position work has been accomplished, taking care of the first step in the snatch and clean progressions. They are already familiar with the press as well, but this will be included in the jerk progression because its practice in proximity to other jerk related drills seems to improve the performance of those drills. If your gym works differently, this will have to be taken into account.

The program is intended to be used 2-3 days/week. How this is actually implemented in each gym may vary considerably. It should be possible to fit this training into the rest of the schedule at least 2-3 out of every 5-6 days CrossFit classes are being run—most likely on days that contain somewhat briefer work-outs.

Clients will go through the program individually—that is, each client will follow the workouts in order until completed. This means that on any given day, your clients may be doing several different drills. If these drills are familiar to you, this shouldn't present a problem. Several clients can be monitored together, and clients who have advanced farther will be able to help clients who are just getting started.

For days on which an Olympic lift is prescribed, clients who have not yet completed the progression can work through all of the related drills they have covered to that point. In this way, they're not feeling left out and are doing something productive with the time while more advanced clients work the lifts themselves.

Clearly trying to dictate multiple series of drills to a group of clients at different stages of their progressions would present a challenge. This problem can be managed fairly easily by ensuring your clients keep records of their training—I suggest having them note on a single easily found page of their training journals (e.g. front or back page) the steps they have completed. This avoids wasted time flipping through reams of marginally-legible post-metCon scribbling. When lift practice is prescribed, each client can simply find the workout that's next in the progression.

These are meant to be drills, not training lifts. Accordingly, there shouldn't be any legitimate weight on the bar, and most clients will be using light technique bars for many of the drills. Obviously drills like snatch and clean deadlifts and certain press variations can be done with more weight, but again, it should be only enough weight to allow the drill to be performed accurately—not as strength work. Each day has about 50-60 total reps—this is a pretty good amount, so rest intervals will need to be kept short to ensure the work doesn't get dragged out unnecessarily. No more than 30 seconds rest should be needed for even the harder drills. However, your clients should be taking a break between sets to ensure higher quality execution. At this pace, the work should be done in about 15 minutes.

The progression drills can be posted somewhere in the gym, or better, you can laminate several copies that clients can grab to keep with them during the workout for easy reference.

What About Advanced Clients?

So now the question becomes, What are advanced clients doing during these practice periods? There are a number of options; which are used will depend largely on how the gym operates. The most obvious is to prescribe more advanced Olympic lift technique drills and complexes to these clients, such as 2 and 3-position lifts, snatch balances, power jerk + split jerks, power clean/snatch + clean/snatch, etc. This is an easy way to keep your clients working as a group; it also improves everyone's training because clients are able to watch and hear your corrections of other clients, which will often be applicable to their own lifting.

Another possibility is allowing your more advanced clients to use this time for the practice of skills they're currently developing, whether related to weightlifting or not. Typically such clients are very self-directed and for such matters are less in need of coaching than simple experimentation and practice.

The Big Picture

Often it's assumed that because of Catalyst Athletics' reputation as a weightlifting gym, our CrossFitters perform the Olympic lifts extremely frequently and have impeccable technique. The fact is, our CrossFit program is completely independent of our weightlifting program, and while, since it is run by me, it does have somewhat more of an emphasis on the lifts and strength/power work than many CrossFit programs, it remains a program intended to develop a breadth of fitness capacities. This being the case, our clients are exposed to the Olympic lifts to an appropriate degree, and are by no means experts in their execution.

In my opinion, the generalist can and should emphasize technique development as much as the specialist—the difference is the amount of time dedicated to each element. That is, while the weightlifter is continuously improving snatch and clean & jerk technique, the generalist will be continuously improving lift technique along with an expansive collection of other skills. Developing an array of skills doesn't mean technical excellence is less important; it simply means that the process of technique development for each skill will occur over a much longer period of time, as it will be continually interrupted by periods of other emphasis.

This is how we arrive at such a program. We intend to teach and coach the Olympic lifts to the greatest extent allowed by the circumstances, expecting a longer process than we would in the type of circumstances surrounding a competitive weightlifter.

Try the program as-is, or modify the template to better suit your application. Commit the time and energy to instructing your clients in the lifts, and they will benefit greatly.

See program starting on page 92

Workout	Exercise	Sets	Reps
1	Mid-hang clean deadlift	5	5
	Mid-hang clean jump	8	3
	Mid-hang clean jump + DL	5	1
2	Mid-hang clean DL	3	5
	Mid-hang clean jump	3	3
	Mid-hang clean pull	10	3
3	Mid-hang clean jump + pull	4	2
	Mid-hang clean pull	6	3
	Rack delivery	5	5
4	mid-hang clean pull	5	3
	rack delivery	3	5
	tall muscle clean	5	4
	foot transition	3	5
5	mid-hang clean pull	3	3
	rack delivery	3	3
	tall muscle clean	5	3
	mid-hang muscle clean	5	5
6	mid-hang clean pull	3	3
	tall muscle clean	3	3
	mid-hang muscle clean	4	3
	foot transition	4	3
	scarecrow clean	6	3
7	mid-hang clean pull	3	3
	mid-hang muscle clean	3	3
	scarecrow clean	3	3
	tall clean	8	3
	mid-hang clean	3	3
8	mid-hang clean pull	3	3
	rack delivery	3	3
	mid-hang muscle clean	3	3
	tall clean	3	3
	mid-hang clean	7	3
9	mid-hang clean pull	3	3
	mid-hang clean	6	3
	clean deadlift	3	3
	clean	6	3
	power clean	4	3

Workout	Exercise	Sets	Reps
1	Press bnk	4	5
	Press	4	5
2	Press	3	5
	Dip Squat	4	5
	Push Press bnk	4	5
3	Press	2	5
	Dip Squat	2	5
	Push Press bnk	2	5
	Push Press	4	5
4	Push Press	4	5
	Tall Power Jerk bnk	6	3
	Tall Power Jerk	6	3
5	Tall Power Jerk bnk	2	3
	Tall Power Jerk	3	3
	Push Press	5	3
	Power Jerk bnk	6	3
6	Tall Power Jerk	3	3
	Push Press	3	3
	Power Jerk	6	3
	Split Foot Transition	5	5
7	Push Press	3	3
	Power Jerk	3	3
	Split Foot Transition	3	5
	Jerk Balance	5	3
8	Power Jerk	3	3
	Split Foot Transition	3	3
	Jerk Balance	3	3
	Split Jerk bnk	4	3
	Split Jerk	5	3
9	Power Jerk	3	3
	Split Jerk bnk	5	3
	Split Jerk	8	3

THE SNATCH

Workout	Exercise	Sets	Reps
1	Mid-hang snatch deadlift	5	5
	Mid-hang snatch jump	8	3
	Mid-hang snatch jump + DL	5	1
2	Mid-hang snatch DL	3	5
	Mid-hang snatch jump	3	3
	Mid-hang snatch pull	10	3
3	Mid-hang snatch jump + pull	4	2
	Mid-hang snatch pull	6	3
	Tall muscle snatch	5	5
4	mid-hang snatch pull	5	3
	tall muscle snatch	5	4
	mid-hang muscle snatch	5	4
	foot transition	3	5
5	mid-hang snatch pull	3	3
	mid-hang muscle snatch	5	5
	foot transition	3	5
	scarecrow snatch	6	3
6	mid-hang snatch pull	3	3
	mid-hang muscle snatch	3	3
	scarecrow snatch	4	3
	tall snatch	6	3
7	mid-hang snatch pull	3	3
	mid-hang muscle snatch	3	3
	tall snatch	5	3
	mid-hang snatch	5	3
8	mid-hang snatch	3	3
	snatch deadlift	5	3
	snatch deadlift + snatch	6	3
9	mid-hang snatch	3	3
	snatch deadlift + snatch	3	3
	snatch	6	3
	power snatch	6	3

WHEN THE OLYMPIC LIFTS AREN'T APPROPRIATE

The Olympic lifts are not for everyone. I'm sure that sounds funny considering the source—most people who don't train in our facility assume that all we do is Olympic weightlifting, even with our fitness clients. This is of course is not a logical assumption, but understandable to some degree based on our reputation.

As it turns out, our fitness clients actually don't do the Lifts extraordinarily frequently. As much as I'd prefer simply instructing and coaching them over anything else, what's appropriate and effective for a given set of clients has nothing to do with my personal proclivities (nor those of any other trainer or gym owner). If it did, our fitness classes would consist of us sitting around watching IronMind lifting videos, eating nachos with triple steak, and drinking cold, crisp, refreshing Arnold Palmers. But alas, I and the other trainers have to actually train people according to *their* goals and abilities.

We have four basic sets of individuals training at Catalyst. The first is our weightlifting team—this is comprised of competitive lifters and a few who are not yet competitive but will be soon whether they know it or not. The next is strength and conditioning clients who are training for particular sports. The third set is our collection of personal training clients, whose goals cover the spectrum of possibilities. And the final is our fitness class folks.

The first group is pretty simple—they snatch and clean & jerk their faces off along with plenty of other heavy related lifts five-six days a week; they sit around a lot between sets and talk about food and the distastefulness of CrossFit.

The S & C folks are easy because they have very clear goals and tend to be more naturally athletic and experienced than many other individuals; likewise, personal training clients are extremely easy because everything can be individualized completely, and generally these folks have well-defined goals, and if not, can develop some with the guidance of their trainers.

The final group is the toughest to work with for a number of reasons, such as undefined or disparate goals, a broad range of experience and ability, and inconsistent training schedules. Generally, these individuals are simply interested in "getting fit" and looking better naked. It then becomes my job as the guy who does all the programming here to determine what exactly fitness is and how best to help such a group achieve it.

Many of you reading this are familiar and may even agree with the Cross-

Fit definition of fitness—personally I was a big fan when CrossFit was using Jim Cawley's 10 traits and aiming for competence and balance among them—strength, power, speed, endurance, stamina, flexibility, coordination, agility, balance and accuracy along with the idea of balancing the capacities of the three metabolic systems—I'm not remarkably excited about the current state of things with regard to definitions and methods.

This is not to say there are not elements of CrossFit that I believe in and implement—there are, and I'm grateful to be familiar with them. However, they are elements from an older and long-forgotten CrossFit, and they comprise only a small segment of what we do.

In any case, these individuals perform strength work, conditioning work, dynamic and static mobility and flexibility work, and corrective/preventative work. Their strength work draws from an array of disciplines, but always relies on a foundation of the big basics: barbell squatting, pulling and pressing variations. There are periods in which they will do more obscure strength movements such as unilateral squat variations and the like in order to ensure stability and balance and provide enough variety to prevent boredom and staleness.

Their conditioning work consists of more traditional conditioning modes like running and rowing of various durations and intensities; interval work with various monostructural and mixed-modal efforts; dumbbell, kettlebell, barbell and other implement complexes; circuits with an array of movements and implements; and short CrossFit-style mixed-mode circuits (with properly executed, rationally-chosen exercises, to be clear).

Within conditioning workouts, they will often use Olympic lift variants with dumbbells, sandbags or other non-barbell implements. Occasionally they will use a barbell Lift variation such as a power clean within a barbell conditioning complex—but with few reps and in a situation that both demands and allows an actual power clean. And never will they use the full barbell Olympic lifts in a conditioning workout as is seen with some CrossFit workouts.

Attempting to curb my circumlocution, let's get to the point: The Olympic lifts are not appropriate for everyone at every time. As I already said, I'm of the opinion that they're essentially never appropriate within a conditioning workout (with the occasional exception of lifts like power cleans at low rep numbers in a controlled and technically sound barbell complex). Additionally, there are individuals for whom the Lifts will simply never be appropriate. My 95 year-old grandmother, for example, has no business snatching and clean & jerking (and no, not even with a PVC pipe—what on earth would that accomplish, exactly?). An extreme example certainly, but the point remains—there are individuals who will seek the guidance of a trainer who do not need the Olympic lifts, and for whom the performance of which is downright silly and dangerous with no arguable benefit. (Yes, the needs of Olympians and grandparents DO differ in kind, not just degree.)

The reasons for this are pretty straightforward. First, the Lifts require a great deal of flexibility that many individuals do not possess, and in many cases, will never possess even with aggressive and consistent work. Without the requisite flexibility, the Lifts are simply not safe with loads that would be effective, like any other activity performed without adequate flexibility. Along these same lines, many clients will have residual limitations from previous injuries that prevent the safe and effective performance of the Lifts.

A reasonable level of strength is also necessary for the Lifts to be useful. Don't argue with me about how beneficial it is for someone to snatch a length of PVC—it's not. Unless it's a temporary stage in a long term learning process that culminates in snatching legitimate weights with sound technique, it's a waste of time and an indication of confused priorities.

Additionally, the ballistic nature of the Lifts means the joints and supportive structures of the body will experience and need to be able to manage high levels of force. The capability to cope with this kind of stress is not innate, and must be developed over time, like most other physical qualities, which arise as a response to certain stressors. Smart programming introduces these stressors and plans the athlete's exposure to them in a manner that provides progressive increases in volume and magnitude with ample recovery time.

In short, when a client walks into your gym, you better have a plan to prepare him or her to perform EVERY exercise they'll be doing safely and effectively, and you better have good reasons for EVERY exercise and workout you expect him or her to do.

Speaking of rationale for exercises and workouts, how many of our fitness clients *need* the extraordinarily great levels of hip and knee explosiveness that demands the use of complex exercises like the Olympic lifts and advanced plyometrics? I can tell you exactly how many—zero. This doesn't mean these things are not potentially beneficial for them if implemented properly, but their absence or presence will not be the difference between fit and not fit. This is much different than the situation of certain athletes for whom the absence or presence of properly implemented Olympic lifts can have significant effects on performance and be the difference between winning and losing.

The idea of training everyday fitness clients like high-level athletes sounds nice and is exciting for those clients, but the reality is that these people are not high-level athletes, and training people is not a conceptual endeavor—there are very real issues to contend with, and very real possibilities of injury and slowed or absent progress when trying to implement inappropriate programming. High-level athletes have years of frequent, well-planned training under their belts that has prepared them for their present training—for a perfect example of this, consider gymnastics and what the kids at each level do. The idea that you can skip over those years of preparation and casually jump into advanced training is horribly misinformed.

It's not simply an issue of safety either, but also of effectiveness. A good example is strength work and programming. Few fitness clients will ever reach a level that requires complicated strength programming like would be seen with competitive weightlifters or powerlifters. Non-strength specialists will simply not get close enough to their genetic ceilings to require such degrees of jiggification. The same goes for tricks like accommodating resistance and similar methods— an adult male with a 200# max back squat doesn't need to be using bands and chains. In fact, not only are inappropriately advanced programming and methods unnecessary, they can be considerably less effective than simpler approaches for such clients.

The previous did NOT say: *Make your clients' training easier.* This idea of adequately preparing your clients for future training and using appropriate methods and exercises has nothing to do with the difficulty and demands of their training, or whether or not they're willing to work hard. While it's true that some fitness clients don't want to push themselves as hard as you'd like them to, there are quite a few who are more than willing to put themselves through surprising levels of pain and discomfort for the ostensible end of fitness (the popularity and rapid growth of CrossFit demonstrates this well). In our entire gym, we don't have a single client who doesn't put forth sufficient effort.

However, within any group of individuals who are willing and eager to push themselves to such a degree, you will be hard pressed to find those who are also able to display the kind of discipline and foresight to critically evaluate their needs, create a rational plan based on these and their goals, and to commit to the necessary training even when it doesn't suit their whims at every given moment.

Typically the kind of work that needs to be done for the sake of preparation for things like the Olympic lifts and other more advanced training is simply not that fun. No one really enjoys things like glute activation exercises or goofy rotator cuff work with infant-size dumbbells. Those with adult ADD may grow bored with their current pool of exercises and want to play with everything under the sun for no other reason than variety. I'm not impressed by the individual who is willing to exercise to the point of vomiting or a loss of bladder control—this is not that unusual. What I'm impressed by is the individual who shows up every day at the gym, does what is necessary, doesn't complain, doesn't look for recognition, does what's necessary outside of the gym to support their training and goals, and continues this process consistently for years.

The idea of smart, appropriate progression is not limited to any particular set of people or training method; it applies to all training, and to all learning, for that matter. We can apply the same principles to weightlifting, strength & conditioning for high school athletes, CrossFit, Pilates, and just about anything else.

This is where the discipline becomes critical—there are times in which what you need to do is not what you want to do. This of course is not to say that you shouldn't be doing what you want—that's exactly what you should be doing. But if what you want is something that requires work, there will be requisite steps along the way that aren't wholly enjoyable.

So what does all this tangential bluster mean with respect to the premise of the article? It means:

- Your fitness clients don't necessarily need to be doing the Olympic lifts.
- If your fitness clients will be doing the lifts, you need to prepare them for it.
- If your clients are going to be doing the lifts, make sure they're really doing the lifts rather than just humping a barbell like a three-toed sloth on Ritalin.
- As a corollary to Number 3, doing the lifts means actually using enough weight to produce some kind of improvement in athleticism.

So let's tackle these points with some semblance of order and organization (to mix it up a bit). But let's do it backwards.

Four: This doesn't mean max weights. In fact, if you're looking to work speed and power, max weights are not appropriate. You'll see the best results in the 70-80% of max range. Take the time to teach your clients proper lift execution and provide them adequate time and exposure to develop technical proficiency before introducing significant weight increases. As I've said about a million times, keep a long-term perspective and accept the fact that proficiency is worth the time and energy investment.

Three: This is essentially the same as Four without the first two sentences. Find ways to teach your clients how to lift properly, and continue demanding excellence.

Two: Make sure you take a rational approach to progress. Can your clients squat, deadlift and press with consistently excellent technique and decent loads? If not, why on earth are you teaching them to snatch and clean & jerk? Do your clients have significant flexibility limitations that prevent them from achieving sound positions and performing the correct movements? If so, they're not ready to snatch and clean & jerk—help them get ready.

One: Determine appropriate exercises based on who your clients are and what they need, not what you feel like doing yourself. Do you want Joe and Jane Fitness to be strong, agile, mobile and explosive? Of course. Will they ever be any of those things to the same degree as a lifetime high-level athlete? Of course not. Do they need to train the exact same way as those advanced athletes, and should they? Of course not. Should they be allowed and encouraged to do things like the Olympic lifts if that's what they're interested in doing? Of course! But it's your responsibility as a trainer to help them prepare for it.

So with regard to Number One, what do we do to work on explosiveness when we've decided that the classic barbell Olympic lifts are not appropriate? First, we do all the typical barbell squatting, pulling and pressing variants to continue developing a foundation of strength. Second, we have myriad (yes, it's *myriad*, not *a myriad of*) options for explosive movements that neither require the technicality of the Lifts nor the potential for injury with improper execution. Any movement that involves driving against the ground and/or extending the hip aggressively fits into this classification. This includes the dumbbell Oly lift variations (preferably power), kettlebell swings (if done correctly), box jumps (that's box jumps, not ankle hops with foot lifts), squat jumps, broad jumps, jumps from the power position with dumbbells or the like, and quite a few other options if you're creative.

What if your clients *want* to learn the Lifts for the sake of learning the Lifts, rather than because they think or have been told they need to in order to be "fit"? Then by all means, teach them and encourage them. But again, do it properly—with respect for long term progress, technical proficiency and adequate physical preparation.

Take the time to evaluate the circumstances and your clientele and make sure you know exactly why you're doing what you're doing. They're paying you good money to help them achieve THEIR goals, whether or not they align with your own, to ensure their training is effective, and to keep them safe and healthy.

ISOLATION EXERCISES

Black and white statements can generally be dismissed as ignorant, if not down-right stupid. Those making such statements may not be stupid—they may just have been persuaded by stupid individuals to not actually think about what they're saying (lots of that going around these days).

Isolation exercises are not functional. Possibly one of the stupidest things that's ever been said. Let's consider why for a moment.

First, to classify something as functional or not, we better understand what the term *functional* means: "designed for or capable of a particular function or use," is how Princeton's online dictionary defines it. By this definition, *anything* is functional; for example, supinating dumbbell curls are wholly functional because they were created in order to train both the elbow flexion and forearm rotation functions of the biceps, and do exactly that.

That being said, I do realize that in the context of exercise, people have a different sense of the word in mind. There is a vague notion of "natural" or multi-joint or similar to certain athletic movements. This still makes little sense, considering that many of what would widely be considered functional exercises have no resemblance at all to any natural movement, and that the variety of athletic movements pretty much ensures that something resembling movement for one sport has nothing to do with another sport. This leaves us with a few extremely basic exercises such as squatting, pulling and pressing variations that could be universally considered "functional".

The point of all this is simply to say that using the functional tag to justify or reject the use of exercises is not particularly... functional. Determining the appropriateness of a given exercise is something that requires knowledge of the athlete who will be using it and for what purpose it will be used. In other words, the question is not, *Is this exercise functional?* but *Is this exercise productive in this case?* Anyone who can look you in the eye with a straight face and tell you that with regard to isolation exercises, the answer is always no, is a moron.

Even if you never once in your entire career use or prescribe an isolation exercise, you should be doing so because you've determined that in all the cases you've encountered, it has not been appropriate—not because you heard on the internet that isolation exercises are only for bodybuilders, and that bodybuilders are unathletic wankers. Neither concept is necessarily true, and more importantly, the mindset that would allow decisions like exercise selection to be made on such absurd pretenses is an enormous handicap for either a coach or athlete.

Since it's essentially impossible to actually isolate a single muscle short of direct electric stimulation or some kind of brain probing anyway, if it makes you feel better, call them *focus exercises* rather than *isolation exercises*—they're simply a way to ensure a certain muscle group, function, position or movement is receiving adequate training within the program as a whole. I'm not sure why this notion has become so repugnant to so many (actually I know exactly why…).

When and Why

The most obvious situation in which isolation work is potentially useful or even necessary is the case of injury rehabilitation, such as encouraging hypertrophy in a post-injury or surgery atrophied muscle. Another is correcting imbalances that are disrupting proper movement and/or creating opportunity for injury. Finally, there are simply certain muscles and functions that are not trained to a great enough degree for certain individuals using "functional" exercises.

A perfect example of this last point is the neck. For athletes such as football players, wrestlers and other combat athletes, neck strength and stamina is critical not only for success but safety. If, as a trainer or coach, you instruct one of these athletes to not do any neck work, because isolation training is not functional and totally uncool, you are irresponsible, ignorant and incompetent and should lose your job. I mean that in the nicest, most supportive manner possible. Personally, I think neck training is good for everyone, whether or not they plan on running into large people or trying not to get flattened against a sweaty mat.

Finally, let's talk about aesthetics. Set aside your puritanical athletic focus for a moment and consider the fact that EVERYONE cares about how they look. Yes, some care more than others and consequently prioritize goals differently. But anyone who says they have absolutely no interest in their appearance is either lying or so enlightened that they have very little time left here on Earth anyway and would have no need to read anything someone like me has written.

There's nothing wrong with this. In fact, trying desperately to prove to the world that you only care about performance, and that anyone who thinks otherwise is sadly misinformed, is, in my opinion, no less narcissistic than of what these individuals are accusing others. Get over it and move on.

Jay Schroeder made a great point once when asked why his football players did curls. Quite simply, he believed that doing curls made bigger biceps, bigger biceps made the players feel good about their appearance, feeling good about their appearance made the players more confident, and that increased confidence made them play better. From this perspective, curls can be considered completely functional for the football player. If it improves performance, who cares how?

So throw in some curls, calf-raises and shrugs if you feel like it, and don't take anyone's shit about it.

Think About It

This article isn't necessarily meant to encourage everyone to start using a bunch of isolation work in their training—it's simply to encourage some consideration of why you're doing what you're doing... or not doing. If you can honestly evaluate the needs of yourself or your clients and determine there is no reason to include any isolation work, there's nothing wrong with that. If, however, there is a need or use for it and you refuse to include it, you need to step back and re-evaluate your perspective.

The internet is abounding with good (among the bad) information regarding neck training, grip training and other similar elements you may consider employing. Spend some time reading and speaking with other coaches and athletes—with an open mind. Just because you hear or see it doesn't mean you have to agree with or use it. But if you don't even give yourself the chance to learn about it, you're going to have a tough time implementing it.

SHOULDER SOLUTIONS

Easily one of the most common problems I'm asked to address by aspiring weightlifters is limited shoulder mobility. This can be one of the most frustrating and protracted processes out there, but its necessity is very apparent—without adequate flexibility, a weightlifter simply cannot support maximal weights overhead in the snatch or jerk. Additionally, shoulder immobility can restrict clean and particularly jerk rack positioning.

This is a simple guide to improving shoulder flexibility in order to improve the positions and movements required by weightlifting. It will not be exhaustive in scope, as there are far too many potential variables to address here, and in many cases, conditions that are best (or necessarily) handled by a professional such as a physical therapist or chiropractor.

Part 1: Correct Positioning

Before any time and effort is channeled into corrective work, it makes sense to ensure that the athlete is actually attempting to achieve the proper positions. Occasionally an athlete will actually be trying to place him or herself in a position that is incorrect or in some manner beyond what is necessary, and consequently believing he or she needs some improvement of flexibility that isn't actually necessary.

Overhead: Snatch Shoulder blades retracted and upwardly rotated. Elbows turn to point halfway between down and back. Barbell over the back of the neck. Head pushed through.

Overhead: Jerk Identical to snatch overhead position with narrower hand placement.

Rack: Clean Shoulder blades protracted and slightly elevated with thoracic spine extended, hands open and elbows held high.

Rack: Jerk Shoulder blades protracted and slightly elevated with thoracic spine extended, bar in the palms, and elbows slightly in front of the barbell and spread to the sides.

Part 2: Diagnosing

Once it's been verified that the athlete is in fact attempting to achieve the correct position, and it is legitimately prevented by a lack of flexibility, we can move on. Diagnosing the actual source of the problem is a bit of a gray area. Most of us are not keyed-in to a degree that allows genuine precision in terms of determining the actual anatomical cause of a given flexibility limitation, especially in an area of the body as complex as the shoulders and upper back.

Fortunately, such precision in diagnosing is unnecessary in my opinion. Most of the time, even if you're by whatever means able to determine that there is a particular muscle responsible for the problem, it's not possible to isolate it correctively anyway (other than by massage or other manual soft-tissue work). Instead, it's typically just as effective, and far simpler, to use more of a shotgun approach that blasts a somewhat wider area containing the problem spot(s).

There are a few basic shoulder functions that we can consider when deciding how to attack the problem: shoulder flexion, scapular retraction and protraction, scapular elevation and depression, and scapular rotation. Each of these play roles in achieving positions required in weightlifting, and generally are interdependent to some degree like most things in the body. This is another reason to not worry about precision diagnostics.

The overhead positions of the snatch and jerk demand great shoulder flexion with full scapular retraction and some degree of upward rotation. The rack positions of the clean and jerk require minimal shoulder flexion, but a great degree of scapular protraction and slight elevation. All require extension of the thoracic spine (or a minimization of its natural degree of flexion).

Part 3: Flexibility & Mobility

There are an endless number of ways to stretch the various structures in question, and virtually all of them can be effective if implemented well. The key to effectiveness is experimentation and determining primarily by feel what is hitting the areas in question and what is not. Generally flexibility efforts will be focused on the shoulder girdle and the musculature that attaches to the humerus from underneath the shoulder (e.g. lats, teres, triceps).

Stretches

Dislocates: With a wide grip and straight elbows on a length of PVC, strap or band of some type, pass the implement overhead to behind your back and return it to the front. Move the shoulder blades up, back and down as you move through the range of motion.

Press Behind the Neck: Starting with a wide grip, press a PVC pipe from the back of the neck to overhead. Start with the shoulder blades retracted and upwardly rotated tightly and finish with them in this position. Gradually move the hands narrower until you're unable to maintain proper positioning, then back off slightly and work at the narrowest grip that allows a solid position with a bit of a challenge. This can then be done in the bottom of a squat to increase the difficulty (Sots press).

Y/I Hold: Lie prone on the floor or a bench holding a length of PVC with a wide grip. Lift the PVC pipe up with extended arms and an extended thoracic spine. Keep the head and neck neutral, i.e. create the correct overhead position at a horizontal orientation rather than a vertical one. Hold the top position for a few seconds, focusing on the activation of the back musculature that is fighting the pull of the shoulder girdle. Gradually work the grip narrower until you reach the narrowest hand placement that allows you to reach the finish position without bending the elbows.

Bar Hang: This is about as simple as it gets—hold onto a pull-up bar and hang. Keep the head pushed through the arms and bring the shoulder blades back together a bit. For those of you who have any amount of chest and shoulder mass, you may find that this position prevents breathing. Hang in there as long as you can and let the shoulder girdle, lats and all that other stuff that wants to keep the shoulder close relax. Keeping the toes in contact with the floor (or a box if extra height is needed) will allow the muscles to relax and stretch more, and placing the feet behind the bar will allow you to lean forward through the arms somewhat to get a better stretch of the shoulder girdle.

Door Jamb Stretches: Stand in a doorway and place the anterior aspect of your forearm against the casing with the elbow bent and higher than the shoulder. Push your chest through the doorway to stretch the pecs. Play with different degrees of elbow flexion and upper arm orientation to find the tightest spots. This stretch can also be done lying face down on the floor and placing the forearm down, and then turning the opposite side of the body up.

Front End Alignment: Extend the elbows and place the hands on a box or similar object at about shoulder height. Keeping the elbows extended, drop the body below the level of the hands and hinge at the hips to flex the shoulders maximally. Leaning slightly back away from the box will help open up the shoulders more. This can also be done with one arm at a time, ideally with the elbow bent. Bend the arm, lift the elbow overhead, and push the upper arm against a door jamb or power rack upright. Stay squared off forward and push the chest forward to open the shoulder maximally.

Overhead Squat: The classic active stretch for the overhead position is of course the overhead squat. Ideally this is done following some preliminary shoulder loosening work. Begin with a wide grip and gradually bring the hands in to the narrowest placement that allows a full depth squat and correct shoulder and bar positioning. A pause in the bottom position will allow some nice active stretching using the musculature of the back to counteract the pull of the shoulder girdle. The grip can eventually be taken in very narrow for close-grip overhead squats, which will in particular force better upper back extension.

PVC Javelin: Hold a length of PVC like a javelin over one shoulder, letting the back end fall down along your side. Reach across your body with the other hand and grab that trailing end of the PVC. With the PVC caught under your shoulder, pull the end up and/or across the front of your body, searching for limitations on which to focus.

PVC Elbow Hook: Place the back of one hand behind the same side hip. Thread a length of PVC through the hole created by the bend of the elbow and your side. Keeping your trunk erect, push the other end of the PVC back, using your trunk as a fulcrum to pull the elbow forward and toward the midline of the body. This stretch can also be done by pushing the back of the elbow against a wall, or if you're flexible and skinny enough, reaching across with your opposite hand to grab the elbow.

PVC Towel Stretch: With a length of PVC in one hand, lift the elbow straight up over the shoulder, bend the elbow to drop the hand down, and grab with your other hand the PVC pipe behind your back. Keeping the trunk erect and the down elbow pulled back with the hand against your back, use the other arm to pull the PVC pipe (and your lower arm) up. To make it easier if you're fat and unconditioned for such endurance events like me, once you pull the stretch tight, wedge your head up under the forearm on top to brace it.

Barbell Clean/Jerk Rack Stretch: Load up a barbell and place it in a rack at the height you would normally use for squats. Place your hands in either the clean or jerk rack position, then partially squat under the bar. Keeping your hands, shoulders and elbows in the correct position, push with the legs to drive your shoulders up into the bar.

Behind the Neck Elbow Lift: This one comes from Mike Burgener. Rack a bar on your back as if for a back squat with a clean grip on it. Keeping the bar on your back and your hands closed around it, lift the elbows as high as possible and push the shoulders forward.

Thoracic Spine: Lie on a foam roller with your spine oriented perpendicularly to it. Roll up and down the thoracic spine, allowing it to relax and extend. You can also simply lie on the roller for an extended period of time to allow the back to bend around the curve.

Lats/Teres: Place a foam roller on a high plyo box, reach the arm up to expose the insertion area of the lats and other local muscles on the underside of the arm, and lean that insertion area onto the roller. Place as much pressure onto the roller as possible rotating your trunk periodically to hit all aspects. This area can also be rolled on while lying on the ground to get more weight on it.

Pecs/Anterior Shoulder: With the same setup described above, roll the insertion area of the pec and its tie-in with the anterior delt. This again can be done on the floor for more pressure.

Part 4: Strength

The primary focus of corrective strength work will be on the muscles that move and stabilize the scapulae from the posterior aspect of the body and the muscles of the rotator cuff. This will be both for the basic advantages of shoulder stabilization, but also more specifically to counteract the pull of the shoulder girdle and internal rotators on the shoulder blades and upper arms.

Press Behind the Neck: This is the same exercise described above as a stretch, but using weight. Eventually work to a jerk-width hand placement. Don't increase the weight so much that it forces the shoulders to round forward and the structure to collapse as the bar starts moving. Focus on scapular retraction and thoracic spine extension.

Push Press Behind the Neck: This is the same as the above, but the use of the legs means more weight can be put overhead. Hold the overhead position for at least a second on each rep.

Push Press: A conventional push press from the front can be used to overload the overhead position if pressing from behind the neck is not yet accessible. This is less desirable, however, because it reduces some of the scapular retraction involved in the movements from behind the neck.

Snatch Sots Press: This is one that may not even be accessible for many until some progress has been made with other exercises. With a barbell on the back of the neck and the hands in a snatch-width grip, sink to the bottom of a squat.

From this bottom position, press the bar overhead. This will require a forceful back extension and very aggressive scapular retraction. If you're not flexible enough yet, don't force this exercise—you will regret it.

Overhead Squat: Not much needs to be said on this one. Do it right, and do it tight. Move the grip in closer for more upper back extension work.

Snatch Push Press: This is the best exercise for basic snatch overhead strength. The key of course is putting the barbell in the correct position overhead—remember, if it's in the wrong position, the right one is not getting stronger. This is a great corrective drill for poor overhead positioning as well—it's an easy way to get some loaded practice of the right way in. Hold the bar overhead for at least a legitimate second on each rep, focusing on shoulder blade stability.

Hise Press: This is an obscure exercise that can be thought of as an overhead shrug. With the bar pressed into the overhead position, depress and elevate the shoulder blades, focusing on tightly engaging the correct overhead position at the top of each rep. This can be done with a snatch or jerk grip.

Jerk Supports: Jerk supports allow a great deal of weight to be held overhead, but caution should be used to ensure it's being held correctly. Again, there is no use in strengthening an incorrect position.

Shrugs: Shrugs are awesome and everyone knows it, even if they won't admit it. They can be done standing with a barbell, dumbbells or kettlebells at the sides, or a trap bar; they can be done seated to reduce cheating with DBs or KBs; and they can be done with a barbell, DBs or KBs with the chest supported on an incline bench to change the orientation of the shrug to involve some scapular retraction along with elevation. These exercises will allow some big weights to be moved, but of course weight should not exceed what allows exactly the movements and positions we're after. It's a good idea to hold the top position for a second or two on each rep.

Barbell/DB Rows: For a basic horizontal pulling exercise to hit the upper back, it's hard to beat barbell and dumbbell rows. In this case, strict pulling with an emphasis on a forceful contraction in the top position is key. Do not let the shoulders round forward or the body to dive to the weight. The elbows can be oriented at different angles for different emphases.

Inverted Row: This is simply a barbell row in which the athlete is flipped and lifting his body instead of an implement. Hanging from a barbell in a rack (or rings or similar), the athlete will elevate the feet to the height of the barbell, keep the body extended and rigid, and pull the chest to the bar, squeezing the shoulder blades together and back tightly at the top. Resistance can be reduced by dropping the feet and bringing them back toward the bar.

Face Pull: Assuming most readers of this publication don't train with cable stack machines, this exercise can be performed with a band or even with dumbbells. With a band attached at face height to a rack, grip the other end and pull the hands to the face, keeping the elbows up and out. The same movement can be performed with a pair of dumbbells if the athlete simply hinges at the hips to bring the torso horizontal.

DB/Band External Rotation: There are probably more ways to perform external rotations than I can count—all are effective if the movement is done correctly. The first of the two most basic variations are lying on your side with your elbow bent to 90 degrees and the upper arm flat against your side. Rotate the upper arm to lift and lower a dumbbell. The other is with the torso upright and the arm abducted 90 degrees from the body (the upper arm horizontal and straight out to the side). With light weight, this can be done without supporting the arm. As weights increase, the elbow will start dropping, so the arm should be supported. This can be done a million different ways—find one that supports the upper arm in the correct position but doesn't impede rotation. This exercise should not be painful. Use a reasonable weight and a controlled tempo.

Dumbbell Y/I Lift: This is the same exercise described previously as a stretch, but with added resistance in the form of dumbbells. Lying prone on a bench or the floor with a DB in each hand, extend the arms completely and flex the shoulders, extend the thoracic spine, and retract the shoulder blades. Hold the top position for a moment before returning to the bottom. This can be done with the arms in an orientation that simulates a snatch grip, all the way into one that places them straight forward. These can also be done with a very short range of motion at the top, moving in and out of the maximum elevation only a few inches.

Programming This Stuff

Obviously which of these exercises are used, how often and how aggressively will depend on individual need and the availability of time and energy. Most of the strength exercises incur minimal damage and can be tacked on to an existing program without much concern. More taxing exercises like the press variations need to be more carefully inserted into the program.

A basic but effective approach is to select 2-3 exercises that address the needs of the athlete and hit them for a series of exposures before re-assessing and rotating to new exercises. For example, the first cycle might use the snatch push press, DB rows and shrugs, each once weekly, and band external rotations daily. For each exercise, the demand should be increased each exposure as tolerated, either by increasing the loading or the volume.

Flexibility work can and should be done in great volumes—as part of the warm-up (assuming the athlete is already warm enough for it to be effective and not injurious), during the workout, after the workout and on days off. Generally speaking, more is better when it comes to improving flexibility. Again, experiment with the stretches and find the ones that work—you will know it when you find them.

BEFORE YOU SQUAT

It struck me the other day while being miserable squatting that for all the talk and writing about how to squat, where to put the bar, how to program squats, there's a lack of talk on what to do *before* you squat. Maybe that's because I'm the only one who thinks it's worth talking about, but hopefully that's not the case.

Step one is to be prepared physically for your squats. This can apply to programming, i.e. don't be trying to do weights, reps, and sets you shouldn't be, but in this case I mean being prepared for the actual movement. Often squats are performed at or near the end of a workout, and if those workouts include things like snatching and cleaning, you're more than likely pretty warm. However, if you're squatting first or after exercises that don't include some kind of squatting motion, take the time to prepare.

Heavy squatting, especially for more than a single rep, is hard enough—when you add an element of discomfort or pain in the movement, your capacity will be limited whether you recognize it consciously or not. The ability to sit in completely and comfortably to the bottom of a squat will allow you to focus on positioning and applying effort to the fullest degree. Pain or discomfort will make you hesitant and invariably force you into different positions. When you're handling big weights, even very subtle shifts in position or your movement in or out of the bottom can cause a failed lift.

The full topic of warming up is beyond the scope of this discussion, but suffice to say you should be consistently doing some kind of thorough preparation work for all of your training. I've previously encouraged you to foam roll during this prep time, and this is particularly helpful when it comes to preparing for squats.

I like to start with my upper back and loosen up my T-spine, which, like in most people, is tighter and less mobile than it should be. If I'm really locked up, I may spend some time after several passes just lying back over the roller at different points and trying to let myself relax.

Next I will roll on my glutes, first with my legs straight out, moving across all aspects. Then I'll cross my leg over my other knee and hit all the hot spots in that lateral area that's typically troublesome. After this, I roll to each side and hit just the crest of my pelvis and around to the rectus femoris origin.

I'll then roll on the front of both my quads together. After a series of passes straight on, I'll rotate so I can hit the VMO of one leg and the lateral distal quad insertion of the other at the same time, and shift back and forth between legs.

From here it's on to each quad alone, focusing in particular on the lateral aspects that tend to get extremely tight and chunky. I'm also sure to make long passes along the length of the quad up to top where I couldn't reach with both legs together. This is where I spend the most time.

Following the quad work, I will hit the hamstrings very briefly since they never give me much trouble, and then with one leg sitting near the end of the roller, I will spend some time on that adductor origin region, which I imagine looks much like the dangerous tangle of cables under my desk. This is usually the most painful area of the session.

Finally, I will hit the calves. This is an awkward region to roll and I don't spend as much time on it as I should simply because I get tired of holding myself up. However, rolling out the soleus in the 4-6 inches above the achilles tendon from back to side is immensely beneficial if you're anything like me and get serious lower leg pain from squatting if my ankles are too tight. This pain is one of the big limiters on sitting in to the proper bottom position of a squat.

Next, I have a stretch I always do no matter what else I do or don't do—the Russian Baby Maker. With my feel well outside my normal squat stance, I lean down and grab the tops of my shoes at the ankles, wedge my elbows between my thighs, and sit my hips down slowly, pushing out against my thighs. Basically, I'm trying to push the proximal ends of my femurs out away from my hips. This is very different from pushing your knees out. In this position, I will shift slowly from side to side and shift my hips up and down. After this I will sit in the squat position and stretch my ankles by keeping my foot flat on the floor and leaning my elbows on one knee, trying to close the ankle as much as possible.

When I'm feeling loose enough, I will grab a mini-band and wrap it around my legs just below the knees and perform a few slow squats, pushing out against the floor with my feet and against the band with my knees (don't push the knees out without pushing the feet out).

From here I'll finally get under the bar (an empty one) for a few squats. These tend to be slow and with pauses in the bottom with a bit of gentle bouncing for a bit more stretching. Depending on how I'm feeling, I may do a few sets with the empty bar or 50-70kg before starting my jumps up to my working weight.

Once you're actually squatting, there are still a few things to consider. While a squat doesn't have the technical elements of the snatch or clean & jerk, heavy sets definitely demand focus and mental preparation. Visualize your set being successful and powerful and generate the confidence you need. Quit talking with the people around you for at least a few moments before you get up for your set. Don't watch anyone else lifting.

Get chalk. With the bar on your back or shoulders, this seems odd, but if you're sweating, dry hands on the bar will make you feel more secure.

Slap your quads, your glutes and your lower back a few times (Use the backs of your fists on your back, or you can lean forward to get a real 2-hand slap on your lower back). I honestly can't tell you the mechanism behind this, but it works. And if it only works because you think it works, it still works.

Finally, be confident and forceful when you lift the bar out of the rack. This will have a significant effect on your confidence for the squat. If you unrack the bar meekly, it's going to feel extremely heavy and you're just going to set yourself up to begin doubting your ability to squat it. Instead, get a big breath, set your trunk solidly, plant yourself squarely and securely under the bar, and drive it up out of the rack without hesitation. Feeling the bar shoot up will remind you of your abilities and inspire the confidence you need.

THE IMPORTANCE OF TECHNIQUE FOR THE GENERALIST

It seems all too common to hear generalists use their decision to not specialize in any given sport or discipline as a reason to not pursue any considerable degree of technical proficiency in elements of their training such as the Olympic lifts. This strikes me as wholly irrational, and indicative of misunderstandings of the role technique plays in the generalist's game.

I have no vested interest in the performances of any generalists other than my own clients, who understand my reasoning for teaching and enforcing continually improving levels of technical proficiency. However, I do have a personal and professional interest in helping people improve their performances, whether weightlifters, CrossFitters, or any other athletes who pay attention to what I offer.

To that end, I'm going to try to make as clear a case as possible for all athletes to strive to continue improving technical proficiency in all movements employed in their training, although I will discuss the idea with respect to the Olympic lifts specifically. The argument at its essence is no different for any other exercise.

Why

The first answer to the question of why would we want to improve technical proficiency is another question: Why not? I quite literally cannot imagine a single reason why anyone wouldn't want to improve his or her lifting technique. Not one. I can think of reasons why one might find it intimidating, time-consuming, difficult... but not without good purpose.

The second answer is simply: To make you better at whatever you do. We use exercises for specific reasons (or at least we should). Proper execution of those exercises ensures maximal benefit. This is particularly true of the Olympic lifts.

The two basic reasons improved technical proficiency will improve the generalist's abilities are 1) Increased reliance on the legs and hips (and improved core to extremity movement patterns) and 2) Increased potential for work capacity. Both of these things are foundational tenets of CrossFit.

GREG EVERETT   115

How

Technique is the method through which force is channeled into the given task; in the case of the Olympic lifts, lifting as much weight from the ground to overhead as possible. A very strong, powerful individual with poor technique will be able to move a considerable amount of weight—we saw this very clearly at the CrossFit Games. But that same individual with improved technique would be able to use that same level of strength and power to move even more weight with even less effort.

The simple fact is that improved technique allows the body to more effectively and efficiently apply its strength and power—the better the technique, the less effort is wasted and the faster the movement is. Regardless of the athlete's goal with respect to the lifts—whether a maximal effort or maximal reps in a given period of time—improved technique will allow more work to be completed via greater loads, faster cycle times, and reduced energy waste. An improved maximal single rep lift is an increase of work capacity in a specific time and modal domain, to use CrossFit parlance; an increased number of reps with an increased amount of weight in any given period of time is an increase of work capacity across any time domain with this particular mode. Both of these things should very clearly be desirable for a CrossFitter.

Objections

I can't think of any objections to what has been stated above, so I won't address any. The only objections I can imagine are concerns about the time and effort necessary to develop technical proficiency. With regard to this, I have a few thoughts.

The only difference between the skill development of a generalist compared to a specialist is that the process for the generalist will be longer in duration, and as a consequence, the level of proficiency ultimately allowable. That is, the specialist will be capable of achieving a great level of proficiency simply because more time can be committed to development, and there will be fewer competing skills. However, the point for the generalist is not to reach the same level of technical skill as the specialist, but to actively and continuously strive for improvement rather than accepting less than optimal technique as adequate—the generalist will benefit from improved technical proficiency just as the specialist will.

Commitment to the process requires a long-term perspective on training—neither expecting mastery in the short term nor giving up when it is not achieved quickly, or at all. Again, the point is not some specific level of proficiency, but continuing to pursue improvement.

Fitting in technique work can seem overwhelming, but it can be done quite simply and systematically. First, recognize how much time needs to be committed to technique development of skills other than the Olympic lifts. No exercise used commonly in CrossFit rivals the technical complexity of the snatch and clean & jerk. The gymnastics-related movements CrossFitters use are extremely rudimentary, the most complex of which is the muscle-up—not even a real skill in gymnastics. The more difficult gymnastics movements CrossFitters commonly work on such as levers and planches are not technically difficult—they just require long periods of progressive strength work.

This being the case, it shouldn't be too much to fit in 1-3 days of 10-20 minutes of technical work on the snatch and clean & jerk—at least for a period of time. Further technical improvement can be developed by removing the barbell Olympic lifts from conditioning workouts until a greater level of proficiency has been reached. This will reduce the amount of counterproductive movement practice you have to correct. Substitute dumbbell or sandbag lifts for the time being. It will be a nice change of pace anyway.

It's Up to You

CrossFit espouses elite-level fitness. It does not promote mediocrity across a broad range of athletic elements. There is no expectation of the generalist to compete with the specialist—he or she cannot. But there should be an expectation and compulsion to continue striving to be better than yesterday.

THE PRODIGAL CHAIN

This is a historic issue for the *Performance Menu*—as far as I can recall, this is its first biblical allusion. This of course has nothing to do with the content of the article itself and knowing this will in no way contribute to the reader's understanding. But it both entertains me and gives me an easy introduction.

The point is simply that as of late, the posterior chain gets so much attention and credit, and the loyal, reliable anterior chain seems to be regarded with disdain, or at least neglected in an undeservedly hurtful manner. Despite this poor treatment, it remains and continues working diligently while the ass-end gets all the play (I won't be as explicit on that particular allusion).

This is not to say (an expression one of my college professors used in infuriating excess while shamelessly demonstrating his vomitous infatuation with romantic era English poetry), of course, that the posterior chain is not deserving of attention; simply that one must balance the training of anterior and posterior chains appropriately, and prevent excessive development of one to the detriment of the other with regard to determined needs.

If an athlete's sport or particular position within that sport demands greater posterior chain than anterior chain development—powerlifters come immediately to mind—then by all means, that athlete needs to train accordingly. However, based on casual observation I've declined to make formal, it appears that many individuals have begun increasing the emphasis on posterior chain training, not with regard to their actual needs, but more as one would alter clothing to suit the day's fashions. This is what we might term *stupid*.

We all know the posterior chain is comprised of the hamstrings, glutes and spinal erectors. The anterior chain consists of the quads, iliopsoas and abdominals—the knee extensors, hip flexors and trunk flexors—basically all the stuff that undoes what the ass-end does.

Most of us value the abs implicitly, because most of us like doing ab work, whether we tell ourselves it aids our athletic performance, or admit that it's simply to look better naked. Many of us end up including hip flexor work in our ab work, intentionally or not, although many who do would simultaneously tell you that you shouldn't do too much hip-flexor work.

The quads have garnered a bad reputation, seemingly because of their association with knee pain and injuries; because quad-dominance in athletes and partial-depth squats that rely largely on the quads have been determined to be potentially injurious, folks have apparently decided that the quads are inherently problematic, as if a design flaw in the human body, the strength and participation in movement of which need to be carefully limited.

The Problem

The problem with all this nonsense is that it's cramping people's athletic development unnecessarily. The pendulum is swinging too far to the posterior side. Encouragement to correct the common anterior dominance is, instead of balancing anterior and posterior strength, creating posterior dominance. In some cases and ways, this may be somewhat of an improvement, but it misses the point by failing to develop the balance that's actually needed—and again, what's needed will vary to an extent among individuals.

The common argument to this is that few individuals are Olympic weightlifters, and therefore don't see a problem with posterior chain dominance. While it's of course true that weightlifters make up a very small percentage of total trainees, these are not the only individuals who need to be able to squat and pull with an upright posture. In a room filled randomly with athletes and fitness enthusiasts, I'd be willing to bet that of all the pertinent and valuable training modalities they're either using or need to be using, the one at which they suck the most is Olympic lifting.

This sucking is due in large part to poor technique instruction and misunderstanding, but also to a considerable degree simply a lack of strength and flexibility in the necessary positions. Addressing these shortcomings very quickly improves individuals' Olympic lift performance. More importantly, in no way does it negatively impact any posterior chain emphasis movements. In other words, if we train it all, it all works. Not a remarkably complex concept. Improved Olympic lifting benefits all athletes, not just weightlifters.

We can find other examples of such posterior chain dominance—or, more accurately, anterior chain underdevelopment—being problematic. The push press—one of the most valuable upper body exercise alongside the pull-up—is overwhelming performed improperly by athletes other than weightlifters. This is of course in part a problem of instruction, but in equal or greater part a problem of the athletes' physical inability to perform the exercise correctly. Athletes whose only exposure to squatting and pulling is of the posterior-chain emphasis variety not only find it odd to dip with a perfectly vertical torso, but find that with any significant weight they're unable because their quads can't manage the load. And then they complain about it hurting their knees, that they can't lift as much, and use this to justify their return to their dropped-chest hips-back push presses and jerks, failing to understand that this is what is truly limiting their lifts.

The CrossFit favorite *Fran* (21-15-9 reps of 95 lb thrusters and pull-ups) is brutal for individuals whose only squatting experience is of the PC-emphasis style, particularly those who aren't conveniently barely over five-feet tall (for these individuals, the difference in squat styles is negligible and the advantage of short levers prevents any real trouble). For those of greater stature, being strong and balanced in an upright-posture squat dramatically improves movement economy and speed. Seeing individuals literally buried under a 95 lb front squat is... embarrassing. Give these individuals some practice in a proper, full-depth upright front squat, and they begin throwing 95 lbs around like full-grown adults should.

To be clear, this is not a call for all squatting and pulling to be performed by all individuals with an upright posture. Posterior-chain-dominant movements are valuable as well. This is simply encouragement for training both—to ensure individuals are strong and flexible through the spectrum of functional movements rather than excellent in some and hopeless in others.

Squatting & Pulling

We see anterior chain weakness manifesting in a number of ways. By far the most common is demonstrated in the positioning of the deadlift and the first pulls of the snatch and clean. I can instruct people to perform the exercises correctly all I want, but as the weight increases, the body will shift itself into the positions in which it's strongest and to which it's most accustomed.

In other words, if an individual's quads are weak relative to his or her posterior chain, we're going to see in heavier lifts, no matter how hard he or she is fighting it, the hips shoot up and leave the shoulders behind during the first pull of the snatch and clean and in the deadlift. There's nothing particularly surprising or anatomically curious about this—the body is simply extending the knee to a point at which the joint's mechanics can make up for the relatively weak quads and shift the bulk of the effort to the stronger hamstrings, glutes and spinal erectors. Along with technique instruction and practice, then, we have a need for position-specific strength development.

Similarly, we're going to see this hip-leading in the squat as well; that is, when recovering from the squat, the individual will naturally and unavoidably extend the knees to a more mechanically advantageous angle while the shoulders (and bar) move very little if at all. This is easily the biggest problem people have with the front squat (and to a great extent the overhead squat). The unloading of the legs because of the quads' weakness places them into a forward-leaning position in which they're unable to support the weight of the bar.

Although it functions to force more concentrated posterior chain effort ultimately, leading with the hips in a pull or squat is not hip work itself; a constant back angle during a pull or squat means the hips are extending in concert with the knees rather than extending to a smaller degree first, and then finishing the movement later. What we want is balanced development to allow coordinated knee and hip extension rather than the see-saw movement of posterior-chain dominant individuals.

Hip Flexors

The hip flexors are a tricky part of this lovely anterior chain. We want to develop their strength and our ability to recruit them when necessary, but we also need to be cautious of the easily-developed inflexibility.

The hip flexors play a number of important roles, but one of the most critical is the maintenance of the positional relationship of the pelvis and spine by opposing the pull of the hamstrings and glutes. This becomes integral to the maintenance of lumbar lordosis in the bottom position of the squat and during deadlifts and other pulling movements. The hamstrings and glutes will, as they contract, rotate the pelvis posteriorly, flexing the lumbar spine and placing it in a structurally unsound position. Activation of the hip flexors in these positions and movements will counter this pelvic rotation and contribute to proper spine and pelvis positioning.

The key with the hip flexors—no different with any other muscles—is developing adequate strength and activation while also developing and/or maintaining adequate flexibility to preserve joint mobility.

Because much of the more interesting core exercises involve hip flexion, and stretching the hip flexors is difficult, uncomfortable and easy to neglect, it's fairly common for athletes to develop problematically tight hip flexors. This then often leads to the reduction or elimination of exercises involving the hip flexors in an effort to combat this increasing tightness. Of course, this just shifts the imbalance in the other direction (sound familiar?). Instead, hip flexor work should be continued, although possibly at a reduced volume temporarily, and flexibility work added to re-open the hips and maintain this mobility. It should be noted as well that weak muscles naturally shorten as a protective mechanism—strength is necessary to support mobility.

An easy way to ensure the hip flexors are being stretched is to force yourself or your clients to stretch them during and after any exercises involving considerable hip flexor action. For example, a set of lunge stretches between each set of glute-ham bench sit-ups, and then another when finished, or possibly the death stretch, will help relieve the tension generated by the exercise. Unsurprisingly, nearly every individual who reports lower back pain during romain chair or glute-ham bench sit-ups—after correcting any positioning errors—in my experience responds immediately to hip flexor stretching before and during the exercise.

Making it Work

I suppose the theme of this article can be distilled to the simple notion of balance. Balance, whether between posterior and anterior chains, or between strength and flexibility, will keep you functioning well rather than constantly bouncing between limitations and over-corrections (and lifting like a wanker). Take the time to evaluate your training, your movement, your posture and your perspective and be sure you know why you're doing what you're doing and whether it truly serves your particular needs or simply the whims or preferences of others.

CROSSFIT CRITERIA

This whole CrossFit thing is getting big. Thanks to the interminable wisdom and foresight of one Robb Wolf—a kind and generous man as long as you don't ask him if he's a runner—I was personally introduced to CrossFit in its public infancy. At this time, the finer details of the theory were still developing rapidly around the very solid yet rudimentary foundation. Gone are the simple days when the affiliates list on the website was only an inch long and prospective clients had to be beaten into submission and forced to train at gunpoint. In the last few years, CrossFit has been evolving so rapidly that the community is in a continuous race to simply keep up with themselves.

Aside from the scale of the operation, CrossFit has been evolving in terms of theory and performance in ways that have provided no shortage of material for passionate debate. One argument that has remained in play and wholly with merit from the earliest days is that of technical performance and the possible compromises that arise from racing a clock.

Technique & Time

Very early in a CrossFitter's training development, there is invariably a clear negative association between time and technique. That is, the more precise the athlete's technique, the worse their times on a given workout. As the athlete progresses, this disparity attenuates and will generally become a positive association—the improving technique brings a new efficiency to the performance, which reduces time. However, as the athlete advances even further, precise technique will often begin to actually slow performance again in a sense by forcing the athlete to adhere to movements he or she is now capable of altering or bypassing. This final stage is the setting for many of the technique-versus-time arguments.

The importance of speed in the performance of CrossFit workouts is so well-established and entrenched that it often assumes priority on a nearly unconscious level. To draw on another relic of first generation CrossFit, Greg Glassman often repeated to the twelve seminar attendees that "Men will die for points." The establishment of the now common CrossFit gym practice of recording workout times on publicly visible whiteboard arose from the recognition of the power this natural competitiveness had to encourage clients to push themselves harder. However, the parameter of comparison was time and so the details of actual movement performance often suffered due to this compulsion to best others' times. With the rapid spread of CrossFit to individuals outside of affiliate gyms and the ostensibly watchful and authoritative eyes of expert CrossFit trainers, debate began to arise among athletes regarding the legitimacy of certain performances being claimed. While in the earlier days of CrossFit, there seemed to be a much greater uniformity among trainers and athletes in terms of acceptable technique for the movements employed, there is now less consistency with the influx of people from different training and education backgrounds as well as those in possession of little if any of either.

Contributing to the problem is the ambiguity of the word *technique* and its application to a broad category of criteria. For the sake of clarity herein, let's establish a more precise definition: Technique refers to the manner in which an exercise, in isolation, is expected to be performed in terms of motor patterns and range of motion; in other words, starting position, ending position, and the movement that connects the two. The key to the usefulness of technique as an evaluative tool is its standardization. If expectations aren't made official, technique remains open to interpretation by all parties involved in the argument and distracts from the core issue. Until those official definitions are published, arguments will remain ongoing indefinitely, and anything I present here is nothing more than a suggestion, although not arbitrary by any means, and presumably not too objectionable.

What are the objectives of CrossFit and how are these supported by a given approach to exercise or workout performance? The answer to this question has the power to resolve the argument by providing clear guidance regarding what constitutes appropriate and acceptable technique. The problem is that there are an essentially endless number of possible answers. The objective of CrossFit is entirely specific to its application—a wrestler, rock climber, fitness generalist, obese grandmother and a CrossFit athlete each have unique demands, expectations and goals, and these are what drive the implementation and consequently the standards of performance. The critical point here is that CrossFit, like any other training methodology or individual exercise, must be evaluated within its given context.

The Limitations of Work & Power

One of the recent changes in CrossFit theory has been the increasing emphasis on work capacity as the measure of fitness, often to the point of obscuring other important details. The detail most commonly neglected in the pursuit of power and work capacity is, of course, movement technique.

Formerly the presented definition of fitness was far more complex and inclusive. This original definition consisted of four parts that together described the state of fitness. The first part dictated that fitness required balanced development of the ten physical elements as defined by Jim Cawley of Dynamax: Strength, power, speed, endurance, stamina, flexibility, agility, balance, accuracy and coordination. The second part was the expectation that the fit individual would be capable of outperforming on average the unfit person in any conceivable physical task. The third part was the notion that fitness resided at the opposite end of sickness on a continuum of health and was essentially super-wellness. Finally, fitness was the balanced capacity of the phosphagen, glycolytic and oxidative metabolic pathways. These four parts created a partially redundant but extremely clear definition of fitness; nowhere within was the idea of work capacity explicitly mentioned. However, improved work capacity and power output were unavoidable if these standards of fitness were met. In other words, the qualities themselves have not changed—only their place in the discussion—but this has been sufficiently confusing.

The term *work* in physics is very specific and differs considerably from the word's common usage, essentially synonymous with *effort*. Instead of the restrictive idea of work, what we should be concerned with is this relationship of effort and productive movement. If we subscribe to the precise physics definition of work and consider improving work capacity and power output as the goals of fitness, the technical performance of exercises and workouts will differ considerably from the manner in which they will be performed if instead of *work* capacity we consider *productive effort* capacity. It will differ further if in addition to productive effort capacity we evaluate the training within the framework of the various elements defined by the earlier definition of fitness, as well as with regard to the needs and goals of each individual.

The Practical Implications

With the shift of emphasis from the original definition of fitness to the improvement of work capacity has come reduced attention to the multitude of aspects that conspire to produce the fitness we're ostensibly pursuing. For perspective, a simple question can be asked: If we could develop better work capacity and power output with exercises such as leg extensions and preacher curls, would we choose this approach over the present one? If we agree the answer is no (If you don't, you can stop reading now), we must value the movements themselves for reasons other than their ability to help us improve work capacity alone. These reasons are myriad, and vary among athletes and training sessions, but can generally be contained within the category of functional value in the mechanical sense rather than the metabolic sense. If we were able to somehow produce improvements in work capacity and power output with curls and leg extensions, we would still lack the motor skills to express those characteristics in the most meaningful, productive ways.

We select movements based on their functional value; that is, we select the squat not because of its potential for work and power output, but because of the motor qualities that train the body to move in a manner conducive to healthy life and performance in sport. That these motor patterns are also capable of producing more work than their isolation exercise counterparts is interesting but coincidental. Work capacity and power output improvements are to a large degree specific to the movements with which the training effects are attained.

Work and power are useless terms in the absence of a medium—the medium through which these physical abilities are expressed is movement. That being the case, consideration of either without a parallel evaluation of the movements producing them tells us little.

Loosely analogous to this problem might be weight loss through nutrition in the absence of training. If we consider bodyweight and body composition our markers of fitness, diet-induced body composition changes may appear to produce fitness. Yet that improvement in body composition does nothing in terms of the motor functions of the body (aside from the reduction in stress on the structures and possible improved mobility from reduced weight and girth), and we're left with a nice-looking body that is still incapable of anything but the most basic functions. In other words, by narrowing the focus too greatly, we may neglect integral components of fitness and may mistakenly shape our methods of achieving it.

If we agree we're training for life and sport, we want the greatest degree of transferability possible from our training to these applications. If we consistently train a limited range of motion of an exercise, it's precisely that range of motion within which we'll excel. If we instead train the fullest range of motion dictated by the interplay of anatomy and functionality, all of the subset ranges of motion will be trained to the same degree along with the range excluded by a limited approach. It's difficult to argue that ability through all potential positions isn't preferable to ability through fewer positions.

Just as we need to prepare for the full range of possible motion, we need to prepare for the spectrum of other parameters such as time, speed, and loading. At present, CrossFit is essentially split into two basic training categories—strength and metabolic conditioning. In the strength category, technique has been prescribed clearly and is generally adhered to without resistance. However, on the metabolic side, technique suddenly becomes open to interpretation, even in consideration of the same movements seen in the strength realm.

Using the thruster as an example, I've witnessed less argument in regard to the finishing position overhead when considered as a strength movement rather than as a conditioning exercise. It's recognized more easily that in order to manage heavy loads, the overhead position must be fixed properly, i.e. scapular retraction and upward rotation with a slight forward torso lean.

What occurs, then, is a gap in ability between the heaviest loading of the strength workouts and the much lighter loads of the metabolic workouts. This of course is less accurate for beginning CrossFitters who typically have lower strength bases and consequently for whom the prescribed weights of the metabolic workouts are much heavier than for the more advanced athlete.

An athlete who can do 225 lbs in a max-effort thruster will still only be using

95 lbs for the thrusters in Fran, only 42% of his maximal effort. If that athlete wants to train, as he or she should, across the entire spectrum of loading and repetition, he or she would be best served by preparing accordingly. As the thruster weight increases, the ability to cycle quickly will decrease considerably and the need to maintain structure overhead for the sake of rest, balance and the inability of the weaker muscles to support the load out front will increase. This seemingly inconsequential detail of overhead position may suddenly become the weak link in the chain and be responsible for significant reductions in performance. This unnecessary drain on performance can be avoided simply by training movements with consistent technique across the range of parameters.

As an aside, it only makes sense to claim that it's inefficient to bring the barbell all the way back into the correct overhead position if we're considering work alone and viewing the movement as nothing more than a method of displacing a load vertically. Efficiency is how well the athlete minimizes effort while moving from the starting position to the ending position of a movement; it has nothing to do with determining where those positions are. We can't say it's more efficient to stop short of the full overhead position because we're now comparing two different movements; if we compared the counterpart segments of those two movements, the manner in which they're performed would be identical and therefore there would be no difference in efficiency.

If we consider a series of repetitions, we may indeed perform more work in less time by stopping short of the full overhead position, but again, that's not increased efficiency—it's an alteration of the movement, in this case a reduction in range of motion. That a movement through a reduced range of motion and more direct path will be able to be executed in less time is no surprise, and it certainly doesn't necessarily improve the training effect of that movement itself. If we reduce the time of performance of the exercise by the same amount of time saved through reducing the range of motion, we've made no progress in power output if we consider that power output to be predicated on productive effort instead of the restrictive term *work*. In other words, we've reduced the effort to a degree equal to the reduction of time and have consequently effected no net change.

A final consideration is that in most cases, including that of the thruster, resistance to such precise performance based on the fear of extending the time of execution is the result of misunderstanding the situation. The final lockout of the thruster is neither a complicated nor time-consuming movement—certainly no more so than the preceding front squat—yet appears to be for many athletes simply because of their lack of experience performing it, and the inadequate speed on the bar when nearing the top to help carry it through to the final position. With consistent practice, the movement will become remarkably quick and demand an inconsequential addition of time.

In the case of the thruster or any other overhead pressing movement, while the final effort to bring the barbell and body into a structurally sound overhead position may not contribute to the amount of work performed, this movement offers clear and genuine benefit that should in most cases override the desire to define exercise technique according to work alone in order to improve power output. Those most immediate are shoulder girdle and thoracic spine mobility, shoulder stabilization, and the balanced development of the local musculature. The question each athlete must ask in each situation is whether or not such a compromise produces a net benefit; the answer will determine how that athlete should perform the exercise.

Fitness, Athletic Training and Sport

The three basic contexts within which CrossFit performance will need to be interpreted are fitness, athletic training and sport. Fitness refers to the pursuit of the most general notion of physical preparedness; that is, no specific athletic goals exist and no particular element of fitness is being given priority other than to establish balance. Athletic training refers to the use of CrossFit-style training for the purpose of improving the performance of a given athlete in his or her sport. Sport refers to CrossFit itself acting as the sport of choice for the athlete; that is, the athlete is interested in improving his or her performance in CrossFit workouts for their own sake and has no interest in training effects in any capacity other than their influence on future CrossFit workout performance.

Performance standards for fitness are the easiest to establish. These standards will be the most demanding of thoroughness because the intention is essentially to train the body for all functional contingencies. The goal of these standards is largely to balance the training effects of the movements employed to satisfy as many of the criteria of fitness as possible. For example, we can't alter a movement to produce greater power output if that alteration considerably reduces another training effect with which we're concerned. In the case of thrusters, for example, this would mean that the rep must be taken to the final proper overhead position. The impact this small movement will have on the time of completion of a workout and therefore the power generated is negligible, while its exclusion may have considerable consequences in terms of strength, flexibility and coordination—arguably far more important elements than power output.

Standards for athletic training will vary somewhat based on the sport and athlete. Workout performance in these cases should be tailored according to the benefits for the sport and athlete in question with no regard to the ability to compare results among the community; athletes need to compare performances in their sports, not in their training. In other words, if the athlete and coach determine a certain standard of performance for an exercise provides the greatest benefit for the athlete, there is no reason to perform it any other way. This will generally mean occasionally relaxed standards of technique—such as stopping short of proper lockout at the completion of repetition thrusters—for greater power output for glycolytic athletes such as fighters. In most cases, however, the standards should be similar to those of the individual interested in fitness: movement performance should reflect the desire to improve as many elements of fitness as possible rather than sacrificing some for the sake of others unnecessarily.

Developing standards for CrossFit as a sport itself is a tricky endeavor. The argument can be made that because CrossFit is in essence a method of producing fitness, the sport should reflect this, and accordingly the standards for CrossFit as a sport should be identical to those for fitness. However, the pursuit of impressive times and feats encourages a relaxation of standards as a means to gain an edge on competitors. Of course, this is ultimately futile—comparison of performances must be made with regard to standards of execution. If an athlete turns in a lower time than a rival because of, for example, a wider push-up hand placement and a consequently shorter ROM, comparisons of the two performances cannot be accurate. This sort of disparity typically encourages the field to conform to the methods of the leaders, producing a gradual deterioration of technique standards that produce meaningless improvement.

Movement should be valued for reasons other than work capacity or power output regardless of the application.

GETTING STIFF: A REVISIONIST APPROACH TO FLEXIBILITY

The reigning notion of flexibility and stretching is that its relationships to both athletic performance and injury protection are positive and linear; that is, as stretching and flexibility increase, so do athletic performance and injury protection. With this in mind, advice from nearly everyone for nearly everyone is to stretch as much as possible.

The actual research and experience of coaches and athletes, however, have failed to convincingly demonstrate this or any other relationship. The research hasn't done much of anything beyond making the subject even more confusing by producing a continual stream of contradictory conclusions, and it's easy to find coaches and athletes willing to supply emphatic anecdotal support for any conclusion you'd like.

Research in the arenas of fitness and nutrition are inherently difficult simply because of the enormous number of variables involved and the impossibility of true control subjects. Studies of stretching and flexibility are no exception. In fact, they offer a number of unique problems in addition to those more universal. Studies of stretching's effects on injury prevention and athletic performance have extremely limited application and are not exceptionally reliable. Anecdotal evidence simply contributes another layer of corroboration and contradiction.

Ultimately both coaches and athletes need a reliable flexibility and stretching prescription regardless of how difficult its development may be.

Definitions

The first step through the sludge of stretching and flexibility is to clearly understand the terminology involved. Often the definitions of flexibility and related terms are remarkably flexible. Unfortunately, the degree of flexibility of a term's meaning is proportional to the term's usefulness: The less precise the definition, the less useful the term. To avoid confusion, we're going to clearly define a few terms for the purposes of this discussion.

Flexibility: The degree to which a muscle can be extended beyond its resting length, which will have a positive relationship with the range of motion of the associated joint(s).

Range of Motion: The degree to which the body can move about a given joint.

Stretching: The set of several methods of increasing flexibility.

Hypermobility: More often called Joint Hypermobility. Decreased joint integrity and excessive possible joint movement as a result of congenitally defective connective tissue development.

Acquired Hypermobility: Non-congenital joint hypermobility arising from injury or joint abuse.

Minimal Flexibility: The minimal degree of flexibility required to properly achieve and maintain specified positions and ranges of motion.

Optimal Flexibility: The degree of flexibility for a particular pursuit that allows the greatest performance and provides the greatest injury protection possible.

Hypoflexibility: Flexibility to a degree short of minimal flexibility.

Hyperflexibility: Flexibility to a degree beyond optimal flexibility.

The terms stretching and flexibility are often used interchangeably in reference to research. For reasons that will become clearer as we progress, this is a serious mistake: they are not the same thing. The terms hypermobility and hyperflexibility are also often used synonymously, but they are not the same condition, and the distinction between the two is only somewhat less crucial than between stretching and flexibility. Hyperflexibility refers exclusively to muscle characteristics: more specifically, a muscle's capacity to be lengthened beyond what has been determined to be its ideal maximum length. Hypermobility, whether congenital or acquired, refers to the joint structure and the excessive possible motion and diminished integrity thereof. The reasons for my insistence on clearly distinguishing the two will become more apparent later.

The Research

Relatively little research on the effects of stretching and flexibility on injury prevention and athletic performance exists. That which does exist provides conclusive evidence of virtually nothing. Particularly in the realm of injury prevention, the research demonstrates little other than that it's nearly impossible to conduct useful, reliable and broadly applicable research of this nature.

Studies can be categorized according to their focus on the contributions of either stretching or flexibility to either injury prevention or athletic performance. It's important here to reiterate the distinction between stretching and flexibility:

stretching is an activity typically employed as a means to increase flexibility; flexibility is the actual capacity for a muscle to extend beyond its resting length, which is associated with the range of motion of the body about the corresponding joint or joints. They are absolutely not the same thing.

The structure of studies and the wording of their conclusions are critical. For example, we cannot misinterpret a study that compared the injury rates of two groups, one who stretched and one who didn't, that concluded that stretching was associated with decreased rate of injury to mean that increased flexibility reduces the risk of injury. Nor can we misinterpret a study concluding that increased flexibility improved a certain aspect of performance in a certain group of athletes to mean that stretching improves athletic performance. And we cannot misinterpret a study that determined stretching was associated with any effects on injury prevention or performance to mean that all types of stretching will produce the same effects. We must be extremely careful to use the data and conclusions of studies for exactly what they are and nothing more, provided of course that we deem the studies reliable at all.

Let's consider a varied sample of the available research.

A two-year cohort study of over 100 high-level soccer players, Gaelic football players and hurlers determined that "flexibility scores were not found to be significant predictors of injury."[1] An RCT study with about 1500 army recruits for 12 weeks had the test group perform pre-exercise static stretching, while the control performed no stretching. Both groups performed a warm-up prior to stretching and/or exercise. The researchers concluded that "a typical muscle stretching protocol performed during pre-exercise warm-ups does not produce clinically meaningful reductions in risk of exercise-related injury in army recruits."[2]

A study similar to the last of about 300 military trainees, in which the test group performed three hamstring stretching sessions in addition to the normal PT program through which both they and the control group went, concluded that "the number of lower extremity overuse injuries was significantly lower in infantry basic trainees with increased hamstring flexibility."[3] A cohort study of Belgian soccer players during a single season determined that "players with an increased tightness of the hamstring or quadriceps muscles have a statistically higher risk for a subsequent musculoskeletal lesion"[4] A study of a Division III collegiate football team comparing the injury rates of players during two successive seasons, during the second of which the players added static stretching prior to training, found that there was an "association between the incorporation of a static stretching program and a decreased incidence of musculotendinous strains."[5]

An epidemiological study of military personnel data cited both low and high degrees of flexibility as factors for injury risk.[6]

It has been demonstrated that passive stretching may temporarily disrupt nerve function, resulting in diminished force production capacity and delayed re-action to proprioceptive input.[7] This means the possibility of slightly less strength and power and greater injury risk if passive stretching is performed immediately prior to activity. A study using college sprinters similarly found that sprinting speeds following passive stretching were reduced.[8] Another study found that vertical jump height diminished immediately following passive stretching.[9] Research regarding flexibility and running economy—cardiovascular efficiency—hasn't generated consistent conclusions. A study of sixteen powerlifters concluded that increased flexibility improved bench press performance over time.[10]

The Bottom Line

These are just a few of maybe a hundred studies. While not an exhaustive sampling, it is accurately representative of the existing research and should help make clear its overall inconclusiveness.

Studies regarding flexibility and injury risk have almost invariably attempted to demonstrate infinitely linear relationships. In other words, they have sought to show that increasing flexibility or the practice of stretching either increases, decreases or doesn't affect the risk of injury, and that this relationship is the same regardless of the degree of flexibility. But what if the relationship—if there even is a relationship—isn't linear? What if there are static points along the plot of increasing flexibility at which the relative relationship suddenly shifts in terms of its rate of change or even direction?

There is also a great deal of variation among existing studies in terms of purpose, subjects of measurement and evaluation, the methods of measurement and evaluation, the subjects, the types of activities, the frequency and intensity of the activities, the duration of the study, and, possibly most important, there is enormous variation in the actual stretching protocols prescribed to the test subjects or studied retrospectively. Some studies focus merely on the presence or absence of any type of stretching in an athlete's training, some focus on the incorporation of a defined stretching protocol—which may or may not align with what we deem appropriate—and others focus exclusively on the degree of flexibility possessed by the athletes regardless of the methods employed to obtain it. These are all very different things and the associated data communicate very different messages.

On average, studies undertaken in an effort to determine the effects of flexibility and stretching on athletic performance are more useful than their injury counterpart studies: these studies more often focus on the given intervention's effects on specific physiological characteristics, such as those cited above regarding the effects of pre-activity static stretching on strength and power production.

Ultimately, there has been one unequivocal conclusion generated by the existing research: Pre-activity static stretching has the potential to negatively affect factors of athletic performance such as strength and proprioception. This conclusion is transferable to the realm of injury prevention because a reduction of normal strength and proprioception obviously both subject an athlete to a greater risk of injury.

Some Biomechanics

Let's briefly indulge in some biomechanics to illustrate some of the most important aspects of optimal flexibility. The spine is a vertical stack of bone segments that articulate on cartilaginous disks. In its normal, stable position, it curves through lordosis in the lumbar region and kyphosis in the thoracic region. In this naturally curved position, compressive forces are balanced over the surfaces of the vertebrae and intervertebral disks. Maintenance of these curves provides the greatest possible structural integrity, while shifting of them transfers increased pressure either ventrally or dorsally to smaller areas of the vertebrae and disks, reducing structural integrity and increasing the risk of damage. Additionally, the spinal erectors' mechanical disadvantage is exaggerated when the lower back loses its lordotic curve—back strength is greatest with the spine in its normal curvature.[11]

The majority of back injuries involve the vertebrae L4 to S1—the point at which the spine and pelvis join.[12] The primary reason is pervasive hip extensor and flexor inflexibility, which prevents proper spinal curvature in anything but an upright position and results in hypermobility of the lumbar spine, which must compensate for the lack of pelvic rotation during body flexion.

Flexion and extension can occur at both the hips and the lower spine. Differentiating between the two movements is remarkably difficult for many people. When I ask my clients to point to their hips, their fingers nearly invariably land on the iliac crests of their pelvises—our sense of anatomy has been distorted by idiomatic English. The hip is the joint of the femur and the pelvis, well below the bony ridges we mistakenly refer to as our hips. Were I to draw a line around the circumference of their bodies at this point, it would be right around the L4 – S1 vertebrae—the joint of the spine to the pelvis.

Public education regarding lifting technique centers on the trite, oversimplified instructions to lift with the legs. But employing the legs in a lifting motion does not necessarily place the back in a biomechanically sound position as the technique ostensibly intends. The ineffectiveness of this advice is related to the misunderstanding of the involved joints as described above.

The lack of distinction between the back and hips becomes problematic during any movement involving bending at the waist ("waist" for our purposes referring to the area comprised of the lumbar spine and hip joints). When the torso changes position relative to the legs, as it does when we squat or lean over to pick something up, little or no control is exercised by the average person regarding at which joint this flexion occurs. This results in the bulk of the work being performed by the joints offering the least resistance—in most cases, the lumbar spine.

This is the primary source of the acquired lumbar hypermobility mentioned earlier. If the pelvis is not allowed to rotate adequately by tight hip extensors, the lower back must hyperflex, reducing or even reversing the natural lordotic arch. It should be easy to see how the frequent repetition of this movement over many years can result in serious laxity in the lumbar spine, all while enabling the hip extensors—unusually resistant to stretching as it is—to grow even tighter.

No matter how strong your spinal extensors are, their activation across a hypermobile spine simply cannot overcome the far greater strength and relative mechanical advantage of the hip extensors. This means that strengthening of the spinal extensors, while absolutely integral to resolving this problem, cannot be considered a solitary solution—it must be accompanied by increased hip extensor flexibility. Nor is the problem resolvable simply by "fighting" the stubbornly static pelvis position while performing the motions during which the problem arises. Direct hip extensor stretching is an absolute requirement.

The best illustration of this—partly because it's the most common situation in which this "fighting" is posited as an independent solution—is the squat. As the depth of the hips increases during a squat, the angle of the back relative to the upper legs decreases, demanding lengthening of the hip extensor musculature. If these extensors are not adequately flexible, they will pull the pelvis with them, leaving the lumbar spine to absorb the remaining necessary flexion. No amount of fighting with the strength of the mechanically disadvantaged spinal erectors over a hypermobile spine will defeat the strength and relative mechanical advantage of short, tight hip extensors.

The idea that improper squat positioning due to inflexibility can be fixed by nothing more than doing squats to only the greatest depth at which lordosis can be maintained and then attempting to incrementally increase that depth over time while maintaining lordosis is not sound. While squatting will increase strength in both the spinal extensors and hip extensors, this ratio of strength and mechanical advantage will remain constant, resulting in no net improvement of the spinal extensors' ability to fight the hip extensors. Compounding the problem is the limited range of motion, which will encourage further shortening of the hamstrings. (This is not to say that performing strength or other movements is not at all effective for improving mobility—simply that it is not a standalone method.)

And now another joint gets involved: the knee. When performing a proper, full range of motion squat, the knees are not subjected to any excessive degree or unusual type of force. The squat is an entirely natural movement and position for the human body, and, performed properly, will fortify the structures and abilities of the body, not harm them. That doesn't mean, however, that all variations of the squat are equally beneficial or without risk. If a squat is stopped short of full depth, undue stress is placed on the knees.

In a properly-positioned full-depth squat (hips below the knees), tension in the hamstrings balances the forces on the knee joint by opposing the force of the quadriceps. If the depth of the squat is not sufficient to generate this hamstring tension, the tension of the quadriceps on the knee is disproportionately great, resulting in potentially damaging shear force.[13]

In short, as a method of attaining adequate flexibility for proper movement and position in the squat, the protocol of squatting only to the depth at which lordosis can be maintained and attempting to incrementally increase that depth over time is ineffective at best and potentially harmful at worst. The protocol must include additional flexibility work.

Some Finer Points

My explanation to many of my clients that they have hypoflexible hip extensors, hyperflexible spinal extensors, and hypermobile lumbar spines is often countered by complaints of lower back tightness, and insistence that their spinal extensors must therefore be stretched and their abdominals strengthened. But the naming of tight spinal extensors as the cause of lumber spine tightness is commonly erroneous. More often than not, the actual source of their discomfort is a combination of tight hip flexors or hip extensors, or a combination of the two.

The psoas is a hip flexor that inserts with the iliacus on the femur, originating on the inferior thoracic and lumbar vertebrae. Tension in the muscle pulls these vertebrae toward the leg, resulting in an exaggeration of the lumbar curve called hyperlordosis and the associated feeling of a tight lower back. The rectus femoris originates on the pelvis rather than the spine, but tension anteriorly rotates the pelvis, having a similar effect as tight psoas by hyperextending the lumbar spine.

Responding as is typical to this condition by stretching the lower back and performing more abdominal—or worse, hip flexion—work compounds the problem by reducing the stabilizing pull of the spinal extensors, strengthening the hip flexors without also lengthening them, and increasing the mobility of the likely already hypermobile lumbar spine, exacerbating existing hyperlordosis and the feeling of back compression.

If the hip extensors are also tight, the summation of their tension on the pelvis and the tension of the psoas on the lumbar vertebrae further exaggerates the compression of the lumbar spine. In this case, posture may actually appear correct in terms of pelvic rotation and spinal curvature because of the balance of anterior and posterior tension. But while the position is normal, the amount of compressive force on the spine is not.

It's critical to be aware of what is and isn't actually tight, and to stretch and strengthen accordingly.

Flexibility and Stretching: The Revised Version

It's my contention that the relationship of flexibility to both injury and performance describes a modified bell curve; that is, both hypoflexibility and hyperflexibility increase the risk of injury and may limit performance. However, in close proximity to the apex representing optimal flexibility—the degree of flexibility associated with the least risk of injury and the greatest performance—hypoflexibility is associated with greater injury risk and greater performance inhibition than is hyperflexibility.

Evidence that has shown stretching to be associated with increased injury rates can be explained by improper flexibility programming and implementation. In short, the increased rates of injuries were due to joint instability or muscle damage caused by improper stretching or from the negative effects of pre-activity static stretching—not a state of hyperflexibility. The majority of studies testing whether or not stretching reduces the risk of injury have involved pre-activity static stretching, which, as mentioned earlier, increases injury risk regardless of a subject's flexibility. Additionally, stretching is an activity that very few people do correctly, exposing their connective tissue to potentially damaging stress, as we'll discuss in greater detail in the next issue.

Another part of my resistance to believing hyperflexibility to be the cause of increased injury rates in these studies is the simple fact that I have met extremely few individuals, athletes or otherwise, who could be considered hyperflexible. In my experience, the vast majority of people—including long-time, competitive athletes—are actually surprisingly inflexible, and, more importantly, possess unbalanced degrees of flexibility among joints. They are unable to properly achieve positions and ranges of motion demanded by their sports, and are therefore accurately described as hypoflexible, not hyperflexible as careless interpretations of stretching studies may suggest.

Some research, like the powerlifter study cited previously, has demonstrated improved performance over time with increased flexibility of the athletes. But these results are very specific to conditions in the study: they don't demonstrate a reliable linear relationship between flexibility and strength, for example. More likely, the athletes in question were hypoflexible to the point of impeded performance, and the flexibility training they performed as test subjects simply reduced that impediment. There is no evidence that further increasing their flexibility would have continued improving their performance.

It's important to understand the difference between reducing or eliminating a performance-limiting factor and actually improving performance. It's also important to visualize this trend on the bell curve described previously and note that past the apex, the increasing flexibility that initially improved performance may begin to harm it instead. In terms of athletic performance, optimal flexibility will not improve in any dramatic manner strength, power, speed or any other physiological capacity. It will simple eliminate hypoflexibility-related performance limitations. If those limitations in a particular athlete are extraordinarily great, however, the improvement in performance gained from increased flexibility may be dramatic.

Requirements

One of the key parameters necessary to developing a proper stretching prescription is an athlete's flexibility demands. There are two categories of flexibility requirements—universal and sport-specific. That is, there is a set of positions and ranges of motion that can be considered requisite to functional, healthy human life, and these obviously apply to everyone. And then there is a set of positions and ranges of motions that are defined by the demands of your chosen athletic pursuits. The degree to which your sport-specific requirements differ from the universal requirements is dependent on the unique demands of your sport.

All athletic activity involves movement and the attainment and sometimes maintenance of certain positions (e.g. static holds in gymnastics). Some sports demand those things in the presence of significant loading or forces far exceeding bodyweight. Sport-specific positions may be functional, reflective to varying degrees of some of our universal positions and movements, while others may be wholly non-functional in this sense.

For example, a flare in gymnastics is a movement demanding of a high degree of flexibility, but it is not functional in the fundamental sense of the word—it's not a movement the human body would ever need to perform in the course of practical existence. A squat, on the other hand, is found in numerous variations in many sports, but also epitomizes functionality in more than one respect.

The reason this idea is important is that when determining your flexibility requirements, you need to first recognize and understand the demands of your existence and their demands of flexibility. In most cases, your sport-specific flexibility requirements will involve a greater degree of flexibility than the universal requirements, but this is not a rule without exception. If you do nothing more than run, for example, you have relatively little demand for athletic flexibility; your sport requires a very limited range of motion of all joints. On the other end of the spectrum are sports like gymnastics and Olympic weightlifting, which demand movement and the control of great resistance through ranges of motion beyond those found in the universal requirements.

The manner in which optimal flexibility improves athletic performance also varies greatly depending on your sport, but more importantly, on its relation to your previous flexibility status. As I suggested earlier in reference to the powerlifters whose bench press performance improved with the incorporation of stretching into their training, optimal flexibility is not technically a performance enhancer, but an impediment reducer. This is important to keep in mind when considering the flexibility-injury-performance curve: increasing flexibility will increase performance and decrease risk of injury if you are presently hypoflexible. But that trend will not continue indefinitely. Beyond the apex of the curve representing optimal flexibility, the trend prior will invert, and it's likely that increasing flexibility will increase the risk of injury and decrease performance.

My focus within the context of injury protection is connective tissue injury.

That said, I don't disregard strains entirely. A severe enough strain can cause long term or permanent deformity and compromise function. But I would argue that strains of that severity are rarer and more difficult to incur than connective tissue injuries. My primary concern is actually not severe, acute injuries, but long term or even permanent damage to ligaments and joint structures. More specifically, my focus within the context of joint structure injury is cumulative connective tissue damage, which, in my opinion, is far more insidious than even fairly severe acute injury.

For example, if you rupture your ACL, you will most likely notice. The condition is relatively easy to diagnose reliably, and surgery to repair the rupture and subsequent rehabilitation seem to be fairly successful. On the other hand (or leg), consider gradual loosening of knee ligaments due to some unspecified activity repeated regularly over a long period of time. No acute injury and its associated sudden pain, noise or unnatural joint movement exists to alert you of a problem that you can then address; the minutely incremental lengthening of the ligaments is completely unnoticeable day to day, and it therefore continues unnoticed until an acute injury, facilitated by this condition, occurs and suddenly draws your attention to your unusual joint laxity.

By this point, the ligaments are probably going to stay stretched. Reattaching a ligament is one thing—making a ligament shorten is another. Thermal capsulorrhaphy—surgical application of heat to the joint capsule to cause microscopic restructuring and subsequent tightening of the joint might work. Of course it also poses the risks of motor nerve damage, over-tightening, and burns to a degree beyond reconstruction. The only practical solution to joint laxity is preventing it.

Universal Flexibility Requirements

The universal flexibility requirements are simple and few, but not necessarily easy to achieve. The first and second requirements are the abilities to maintain proper lumbar spine extension through the entire range of motion of two movements: a full-depth squat and hip flexion to a minimum of 90 degrees relative to the legs. The third requirement is the ability to achieve a proper overhead position.

Limited mobility in the shoulder girdle and thoracic spine are a commonly overlooked cause of lower back injuries and pain. If the shoulders are unable to open fully (extend the arms vertically), the overhead position is not actually overhead. Therefore, when attempting to lift the arms overhead, the lumbar spine tends to hyperextend, rotating the torso backward to allow the arms attached to the partially opened shoulders to extend vertically. The ability to fully open the shoulder, then, is integral to long-term functionality and injury prevention.

The Bottom Line

In short, a flexibility prescription is concerned with two areas: injury prevention and performance impediment elimination. In terms of injury prevention, the goal is to reduce the likelihood of musculotendinous, ligamental or other injuries, with its primary focus being the reduction of potentially damaging stress to connective tissue and the maintenance of joint integrity. In terms of performance, the goal is to eliminate any impediments arising from either hypo- or hyperflexibility.

In order to achieve these goals, the prescription must be predicated on determined flexibility requirements, of which there are two types: universal and specific. Universal requirements are those that apply to everyone; specific requirements are unique to each sport or activity and must be determined individually for each athlete. The protocol must employ proper stretching methods that achieve the desired goals but do not at all threaten joint integrity or performance.

Endnotes

1 Watson AW. Sports injuries related to flexibility, posture, acceleration, clinical defects, and previous injury, in high-level players of body contact sports. Int J Sports Med. 2001 Apr;22(3):222-5. http://www.ncbi.nlm.nih.gov/entrez/query.fcgi?cmd=Retrieve&db=pubmed&dopt=Abstract&list_uids=11354526&query_hl=10&itool=pubmed_docsum

2 POPE, R. P., R. D. HERBERT, J. D. KIRWAN, and B. J. GRAHAM. A randomized trial of preexercise stretching for prevention of lower-limb injury. Med. Sci. Sports Exerc., Vol. 32, No. 2, pp. 271-277, 2000. http://www.ncbi.nlm.nih.gov/entrez/query.fcgi?cmd=Retrieve&db=PubMed&list_uids=10694106&dopt=Abstract

3 Hartig DE, Henderson JM. Increasing Hamstring Flexibility Decreases Lower Extremity Overuse Injuries in Military Basic Trainees. The American Journal of Sports Medicine 27:173-176 (1999). http://ajsm.highwire.org/cgi/content/abstract/27/2/173

4 Witvrouw E, Danneels L, Asselman P, D'Have T, Cambier D. Muscle flexibility as a risk factor for developing muscle injuries in male professional soccer players. A prospective study. Am J Sports Med. 2003 Jan-Feb;31(1):41-6. http://www.ncbi.nlm.nih.gov/entrez/query.fcgi?cmd=Retrieve&db=PubMed&list_uids=12531755&dopt=Abstract

5 Cross KM, Worrell TW. Effects of a Static Stretching Program on the Incidence of Lower Extremity Musculotendinous Strains. J Athl Train. 1999 Jan–Mar; 34(1): 11–14. http://www.pubmedcentral.nih.gov/articlerender.fcgi?artid=1322867

6 Jones BH, Knapik JJ. Physical training and exercise-related injuries. Surveillance, research and injury prevention in military populations. Sports Med. 1999 Feb;27(2):111-25 http://www.ncbi.nlm.nih.gov/entrez/query.fcgi?cmd=Retrieve&db=PubMed&list_uids=10091275&dopt=Abstract

7 Katagi K. Stretching: The Truth. Ski. March-April 2006: 96-98.

8 Nelson AG, Driscoll NM, Landin DK, Young MA, Schexnayder IC. Acute effects of passive muscle stretching on sprint performance. Journal of Sports Science. Vol 23 Number 5 / May 2005 Pages: 449 – 454. http://taylorandfrancis.metapress.com/(dvs4ow22amtfxx-45mfqeclel)/app/home/contribution.asp?referrer=parent&backto=issue,2,12;journal,12,105;linkingpublicationresults,1:100184,1

9 Cornwell A, Nelson AG, Sidaway B. Acute effects of stretching on the neuromechanical properties of the triceps surae muscle complex. European Journal of Applied Physiology. 2002 Mar:Volume 86, Number 5 Pages: 428 - 434 http://www.springerlink.com/(bz2ey555uqfl-r2atfv4xhq45)/app/home/contribution.asp?referrer=parent&backto=issue,9,12;journal,45,425;linkingpublicationresults,1:100513,1

10 Wilson GJ, Elliott BC, Wood GA. Stretch shorten cycle performance enhancement through flexibility training. Med Sci Sports Exerc. 1992 Jan;24(1):116-23. http://www.ncbi.nlm.nih.gov/entrez/query.fcgi?cmd=Retrieve&db=PubMed&list_uids=1548985&dopt=Citation

11 Baechle TR, Earle RW. The Essentials of Strength Training and Conditioning. Champaign: Human Kinetics; 2000.

12 Baechle TR, Earle RW. The Essentials of Strength Training and Conditioning. Champagne: Human Kinetics; 2000.

13 Rippetoe M, Kilgore L. Starting Strength. Wichita Falls: The Aasgaard Company; 2005.

THE PUSH-UP: WHY IS THIS SO HARD?

One of the things in my life that continually mystifies me is how something as simple and pure as the push-up has become so confusing and impossible for so many people. This is like the exercise equivalent of every adult in the world suddenly forgetting how to walk (yet still wanting to do the triple jump).

This very issue is what caused me to add planks into every day of our introductory class series. I was embarrassed by the inability of people in the gym to do excellent push-ups and decided that the most pro-active approach I could take would be to train them from day one how to do it rather than trying to re-engineer them later down the line when they're uninterested and just think I'm being a dick about it.

The priorities for the push-up as I see them are, in order: correct and rigid posture, including head position; range of motion; elbow orientation; resistance.

First and foremost, if someone can't hold his or her body tightly in a straight line from ankle to ear, they're unable to do proper push-ups. You can kick and squirm and fight this idea all you want, but you can't escape it. You should be able to visually draw a straight line from the ankle, through the hip and through the shoulder at any point in the push-up, and the head and neck should remain in a neutral position—dipping the chin to the floor isn't getting you to the bottom of the movement and only makes you look like a saggy hunchback who is likely incontinent.

This rigid alignment should never change throughout the exercise. Don't push your shoulders up and then later bring your hips up to meet them. This isn't a push-up and it looks weird.

Next is the range of motion. This shouldn't have to be specified after saying "push-up" but there seems to be some confusion surrounding it. At the top, the elbows should be completely extended and the shoulder blades protracted. At the bottom, the chest should be in light contact with the floor. Again, in both of these positions and everywhere in between, the body should be straight and rigid.

This full range of motion in my opinion should take precedence over the degree of resistance. That is, if you can't complete a push-up to full depth from the toes, you need to modify it somehow, such as moving to the knees or elevating your hands. Remember when on your knees, you still need to maintain a rigid straight body—the knees simply replace your ankles in this case. The hands can be elevated on a wall, but the wall gets in the way of the face—you're better off moving the hands to a plyo box or bench so the head can travel without obstruction and make the correct posture possible.

I encourage clients who can do a few standard push-ups to begin workouts with them and move to the knees when needed to maintain the range of motion. This can be difficult on the ego, especially for men, but the benefits are worth any potential embarrassment. No one loads a weight on the bar and benches it halfway down because it's too heavy (well... excepting board pressing and the like); they start with a weight they can move through the entire range of motion and build up from there. Why the push-up (and pull-up for that matter) are viewed differently, I don't know.

I prefer the upper arms to be within about 45 degrees from the sides of the body. This allows the shoulder to move through that full range of motion more easily and naturally. Moving the hands wider and bringing the elbows farther from the sides will usually make push-ups easier for people, but it also limits depth for most people and starts tearing up the shoulders pretty quickly.

The push-up is one of those things that when done well doesn't draw much attention—it's not a flashy feat of athleticism. However, in my opinion, how one performs a push-up is indicative of that individual's athletic foundation, and possibly more importantly, how committed one is to excellence in movement and performance. Sloppy push-ups suggest to me a superficial interest in athleticism and a degree of laziness. Put a little attention and effort into the simple things and it will pay returns in the more complicated and interesting ones.

THE PORTABLE GREG EVERETT

THE KETTLEBELL SWING

I want to address the kettlebell swing in response to an email I got about it. Those of you who pay attention to CrossFit are familiar with the practice of continuing the KB swing overhead rather than the traditional level. The question I got was basically, Why do either, and is there any sort of injury risk or similar with the overhead swing?

Most of the time I prefer the traditional swing, and always with individuals new to the exercise. The point of the KB swing is the explosive snap of the hips. You can get other things out of it, but this is the primary goal and if it's not there, you should probably be doing a different exercise for whatever you're trying to accomplish.

With a focus on this hip action, the KB will rise to chest or chin height easily with no work from the arms and shoulders. Again, this is the point—you shouldn't be muscling the bell up with your arms. Clients new to the exercise should only work at this level until they've mastered the hip action of the swing. Once that's done, overhead swings can be considered an option.

The overhead swing should look identical to the traditional swing in the bottom range of motion—that is, the snappy hip action should not disappear. Once it's completed, you engage the back and shoulders to continue pulling the bell up and back and drive the chest in underneath it.

There are a couple good things about the overhead swing. First, of course, you're involving more of the body in the movement, so it's a more complete exercise. Second, the greater height of the bell means you can easily generate more downward momentum going into the next rep; this means the hips and back must absorb more force and therefore are being trained harder (This of course can also be accomplished with a traditional swing by simply making the effort to accelerate the bell down after each rep, or with partner power bombs). Finally, if you're using the swing as a conditioning exercise, this means more work and consequently more gas necessary.

I have two basic concerns regarding the overhead swing. The first is for the safety of both the swinger and those around him or her. Tired clients tend to get squirrely, especially in an environment in which high volume overhead swinging in a fatigued state is encouraged. I have seen more than a few people lose control of a KB overhead and damn near make an ashtray in the top of their skulls. I have also seen people drop the bells from overhead or nearly overhead and almost take out a neighbor. And I've even seen a complete moron drop a kettlebell from overhead onto cement and snap the handle right off (a few of you reading this know exactly who I'm talking about—his profession makes it even more embarrassing.).

My second concern is simply that often people get caught up in the effort to bring the bell overhead and their hip snap disappears. Instead we get a slow, soft hump with a big upper body effort. I'll say it again—this really defeats the purpose of the swing. And this is why I only like overhead swings for people who are able to do good traditional swings and maintain that hip action when going overhead.

So aside from traumatic head injury or getting sniped by a bouncing kettlebell dropped by someone nearby, I don't see any injury concerns with the overhead swing for individuals with adequate overhead mobility.

Ultimately the traditional swing should be the exercise first taught and mastered, and should be the variation used most. It's an excellent exercise for conditioning the lower back, glutes and hamstrings to volume, improving lower back stamina and stability, and yes, even for cardio conditioning—a series of heavy swings to the chin will get you plenty exhausted without going overhead.

Do both if you want, but do them right, and don't drop them on your head.

THOUGHTS ON THE KIPPING PULL-UP

The kipping pull-up has been a point of vehement contention since its popularization by CrossFit; one camp tells the world it's the only way to create complete elite athletic dominance and will possibly cure all known disease, and the other claims they will fail to develop much of anything athletic but will completely destroy your shoulders. It seems unlikely that any of these is entirely true.

I've never spoken up much either way before, except to express my distaste for the "butterfly" kip, and even that wasn't too enthusiastic, and discuss the pull-up in general terms in other articles. Recently the heat seems to have been turned up a bit and I'm seeing more and more discussion on the topic, focused primarily on the injury potential of the exercise. I've avoided getting involved for a few reasons, not the least of which is that I feel it's an unwinnable war and any opinions I share on the topic will piss at least a few people off. I don't mind this exactly, but I have a hard time not then engaging in stupid internet arguments, so I prefer to avoid setting them up in the first place. But I'll give this one a shot anyway.

First, I will reiterate my dislike of the butterfly kip. Its sole purpose is to serve as a competitive pull-up style (whether or not this is recognized or admitted), and this alone is enough to dissuade me from ever using it, teaching it or endorsing it. The idea of modifying an exercise to reduce effort and increase speed for the sake of beating a clock or another exerciser doesn't make much sense to me. Exercises should have purpose and rationale; for example, a pull-up is a great way to develop upper body pulling strength, scapular stability and even muscular and cardiorespiratory endurance if performed in higher volumes. The butterfly kip minimizes the demands on the very things that the exercise should be used to develop. Additionally, it brings an element of stress to the shoulders and elbows of which the potential for injury is far greater than a more traditional kipping movement. Were I a CrossFit Gamer or some other type of competitive exerciser, I would use the butterfly kip. But again, that very notion tells me it's not a good choice for training, other than periodic practice for impending competition.

The pull-up is such a fundamental, foundational exercise that it belongs, in some form, in the training of just about everyone. Note that this might mean extreme modifications for some individuals—it doesn't necessarily mean that grandma is swinging around on a pull-up bar after her shoulder surgery.

The strict pull-up should be considered the standard from which all variations stem, and it should be the standard to which everyone strives. That is, if you're going to do pull-ups of any kind, one of your ultimate goals should be being capable of multiple strict pull-ups. Variations have their places, but never are they replacements for the pull-up itself.

The more traditional kipping style that was originally endorsed by CrossFit before the advent of the butterfly kip and the CrossFit Games should be considered a totally different exercise and discussed accordingly. That is, if we're talking about injury potential, we can't confuse the butterfly and traditional kip variations—the movements are too dissimilar, and I'm of the opinion that much of the increasing rate of pull-up-related shoulder injury is directly related to the increasing rate of butterfly kipping rather than traditional kipping.

In a properly performed traditional kipping pull-up, after locking out over the bar, the athlete pushes back from the bar into an arc that loads the forward push of the chest through the arms prior to the following rep. This is a smooth, controlled movement; by no means is it jarring or ballistic unless done improperly. There is continuous tension throughout the descent, and the force is fluidly transitioned between horizontal and vertical planes. The loading of the shoulders is neither abrupt nor directed in a way that subjects the shoulder joint to anything it shouldn't be more than capable of withstanding.

The butterfly kip, on the other hand, sends the athlete forward under the bar into the bottom. There is an unavoidable moment of slack and freefall, followed by the shoulders being opened completely in a relatively jarring manner—being pulled closer to straight up from the body rather than stretched progressively with more horizontal movement. In theory this could be controlled more than it typically is, and the movement better guided, but the fact is that anyone doing a butterfly kip has clearly prioritized other things (i.e. speed) or in many cases is simply unaware of any of this and is simply emulating CrossFit superstars.

In any case of kipping pull-ups, adequate preparation is necessary for safety. This is not unique to the kipping pull-up; it's true for any physical activity. Where this becomes problematic often is situations in which inadequate progression exists due to impatience or ignorance. Another great example of this that I've seen many times are middle-aged individuals with no athletic background and extremely brief training histories being instructed to perform huge volumes of plyometric movements. Like kipping pull-ups, plyometrics aren't unavoidably injurious—they just require smart implementation, which involves proper progression, execution and programming.

With regard to kipping pull-ups, if an individual can barely string together a couple of ring rows at a high angle, jumping them into kipping pull-ups is ill-advised to say the least, yet this happens all the time. There is such a rush to get people doing pull-ups (or loose interpretations thereof) that simple, seemingly obvious things like this are often overlooked or ignored.

With new clients at Catalyst, the body row on rings is the initial introduction to the pull-up. This does a few things. First, it provides an opportunity for us to assess a client—it's stunning how weak many are, both in terms of the ability to pull themselves to the rings and to maintain trunk rigidity. The body row is a chance for clients to feel what it's like to really engage the upper back—to retract the scapulae powerfully, feel the lats extend the spine, and feel the shoulders engage to bring the arms back. These things are frequently missing from pull-ups, particularly kipping pull-ups, and even more so when kipping pull-ups are a client's first introduction to upper body pulling exercises. The exercise also begins strengthening the shoulders and elbows and preparing them to withstand greater stresses like what they'll need to manage with pull-ups of any kind.

The next thing our new clients are exposed to is strict pull-ups with whatever assistance is necessary. We use elastic bands at times, but I actually prefer leg assistance. The problem with bands is that the tension is exactly the opposite of what's needed—that is, it's greatest the bottom when the client needs it least, and it's greatly reduced at the top when the client needs it the most. This exacerbates the problem of clients not engaging their upper backs as much as they should, and prevents them from ever developing the strength to do so. Instead, they finish the movement with all arm flexors, a forward roll of the shoulders and a reach of the chin. With leg assistance, the client can instantly adjust to provide exactly as much assistance as is needed. It's impossible to measure progress in this manner, but bands aren't exactly great for this either—the jumps between band sizes are way too large. As long as you keep an eye on your clients, they'll be using less and less assistance. It's quite obvious when watching when they're using more leg assistance than necessary.

Only after three weeks of body rows and leg assisted strict pull-up work do our new clients even get introduced to the idea of a kipping pull-up. This initial introduction involves teaching the basic kipping movement, which more than being movement instruction, begins to help stretch the shoulder girdle in a safe and controlled manner to prepare for the necessary range of motion for a safe and controlled kipping pull-up. The strict pull-up remains the target even after this.

To wrap up what was supposed to be a brief article, I don't believe the traditional kipping pull-up is any more dangerous than many other useful exercises. Like any of these other exercises, though, it demands smart progression and implementation. Kipping pull-ups of any variety are also not substitutes for strict pull-ups and rowing-type exercises. They are a unique exercise that can have a place in many individuals' training—just not the strict pull-up's place.

GREG EVERETT

A MORE CIVILIZED APPROACH TO BLEEDING

The promotion of blood donation is invariably approached from the angle of altruism. Promotional strategies emphasize the need for 38,000 pints of blood every day in the US—a pint almost every 2 seconds—for the regular and emergency treatment of a range of individuals, from cancer patients to burn victims to premature infants (who are in all probability thoroughly adorable).

But what if you're cruel, selfish and uncaring by nature? It turns out there might be some good reasons for you to donate too.

The most common reasons to be found in the research are predicated on excess iron storage. Iron is requisite to human and most non-human life on the planet. In the body, iron's primary function is aiding the transport of oxygen by red blood cells as hemoglobin, but it also plays a number of other roles, including assisting in the synthesis of DNA, collagen, and other protein structures. At the same time, iron poses serious risks to life as a potent pro-oxidant. Because of this, the treatment of iron by the body is remarkably careful: the absorption, distribution and storage of iron is reliant on a well integrated system of protein structures that prevent iron's direct exposure to the rest of the body.

Iron Absorption & Storage

There are two types of dietary iron: heme and non-heme. Heme iron is the form found in meat and is the more efficiently absorbed type (15% - 35%). Non-heme is found in plant foods and is less easily absorbed (2% - 20%), although its absorption rate is more greatly influenced by accompanying dietary factors. Meat, vitamin C and fructose all enhance the absorption of non-heme iron, while soy, calcium, phytates (nutrient-binding protein found in grains) and tannins and polyphenols (both found in tea) reduce its absorption.

When dietary iron enters the guts, it is taken up into enterocytes, epithelial cells lining the walls of the intestine. If systemic iron levels are low enough to require uptake, the iron is encased by the transferrin molecule and distributed through the body as appropriate. Otherwise the iron remains in the enterocytes, which regularly die and pass from the body, bringing the unabsorbed iron along. Average daily iron loss though mechanisms such as sweating, urination, and the regular sloughing of integumentary components is around 0.9 mg (pre-menopausal women may lose an additional 15-20 mg per month through menstruation). These losses are easily covered by anything that remotely resembles a decent diet.

So in theory, this combination of controlled absorption and regular dietary replenishment should maintain ideal iron levels in the body. Unfortunately it's not a flawless system, particularly when challenged by unnatural modern factors.

Nearly all grain foods in the US are fortified with easily absorbable iron. Many people take daily multivitamin/mineral supplements with sometimes enormous amounts of iron. High-fructose corn syrup is used to sweeten nearly every packaged food in addition to soda. In short, there is an epic assortment of variables that can potentially override the body's controlled absorption system and leave us with more iron in storage than we need.

The body has no internal mechanism for excreting excess iron. It simply contains it in protective protein molecules and stores it in tissues, preferentially glandular tissue such as that of the liver and pancreas. In the past, humans did have a way of dropping excess iron—we were full of parasites, creating continuous minor gastrointestinal bleeding—iron contained in the hemoglobin was in this fashion dumped from the body. This constant blood loss was likely the reason we evolved with mechanisms to protect iron and none to eliminate it.[1]

Those of us living in developed areas of the world are now free of the parasitic bleeding that reduces iron stores, but also subject to unnatural foods that are either fortified with iron, enhance the absorption of iron, or both. Over years, this can result in unusually high levels of iron in the body.

So What's the Problem?

The primary problem with iron is its pro-oxidant characteristics: it's very good at helping create free radicals—molecules with unpaired electrons with consequently low stability and high reactivity—such as the hydroxyl radical.

In heart attacks and strokes, the bulk of the tissue damage is actually not due to oxygen deprivation, but instead to the re-introduction of oxygen. When an artery is occluded, tissues beyond the blood's reach are deprived of the accompanying oxygen and begin dying. Necrotic cell death is not orderly—pieces essentially fall apart freely—and this allows the free exposure of formerly safely stored iron. When the vessel occlusion is repaired, whether medically or naturally, a huge influx of blood bathes these broken tissues and the exposed iron, which reacts with the new oxygen. This violent reaction can result in severe tissue damage.

Excessive iron storage may also be a factor in the development of certain cancers such as of the liver, atherosclerosis, reduced insulin production and insulin resistance. The research on which these ideas are founded is—like almost all research in similar areas—not conclusive, but does appear relatively convincing.

Regular flushing and replacement of iron also means the body will have fresh material for hemoglobin and other iron-dependent structures instead of relying on continual recycling. The benefit of this is entirely speculative, but no potential drawbacks seem to exist.

Testing Your Iron Level

If you're interested in having your stored iron level tested, don't let your doctor test your hemoglobin level—this is common but inaccurate method. Instead, ask for a serum ferritin test, which measures the amount of ferritin in the blood. This number is 10 times lower than your iron level; that is, if your serum ferritin number is 70, you have 700 mg of stored iron. Certain individuals may show inaccurately high ferritin levels, including alcoholics and those with infections, severe inflammation, and cancer.[2]

A healthy amount of stored iron is around 500 mg. 1000 mg may be problematic. 150 mg is a safe low-end threshold. Less than 100 mg is indicative of iron-deficiency anemia.[3]

Donating Blood

Getting rid of blood is not hard—there are a lot of people out there more than happy to relieve you of some. They won't even charge you for it.

My own blood donations have been consistently positive experiences. Aside from enjoying scintillating conversation with the lovely phlebotomists and volunteer post-drainage babysitters who like to make continual subtle advances toward my defiant position with the donut tray, I've noticed a significant improvement in energy in the days following the donations. I've also been perfectly able to train at adequate intensity and volume within several hours of donation, despite my repeated and convincing assurances to my concerned caretakers that I would never dream of engaging in such reckless behavior. Performance in high-oxidative-metabolism-demand training will be below average with a pint less blood in your system, but generally donation frequency is limited to eight weeks—a regular blood donation schedule that coincides with a week of limited training volume and intensity could be a simple method of ensuring periodic active recovery in your long-term training strategy.

The bottom line is actually very simple: while the potential health benefits of regularly donating blood have yet to be demonstrated conclusively, with proper nutrition and lifestyle, and with consideration of known contraindications, blood donation poses little if any risk. That being the case, the prudent course of action is to make regular blood donation a habit. The worst case scenario is that your blood helps save the life of some cute little baby and your metabolic conditioning is compromised for a week every two months.

1 Eades, M, Eades, MD. *Protein Power Lifeplan: A New Comprehensive Blueprint for Health.* New York: Warner Books; 2000.
2 Health A to Z. Iron Tests. Available at: http://www.healthatoz.com/healthatoz/Atoz/ency/iron_tests.jsp
3 Eades, M, Eades, MD. *Protein Power Lifeplan: A New Comprehensive Blueprint for Health.* New York: Warner Books; 2000.

ATTITUDE ADJUSTMENT

I do my best to fly under the radar (phrase and advice supplied by Eva T years ago)—to do my thing, do it as well as I can, and let the rest slide off my back. Drama pervades the fitness and strength & conditioning industry, the flame oxidized by the cheapness of words in an online world with little consequent and virtually no accountability. It's an epic and unending battle among keyboard warriors.

Last weekend, Aimee and I traveled up to Chico, CA to give a weightlifting clinic at NorCal Strength & Conditioning, the gym now owned and run stupendously by my former partners in the business, Robb Wolf and Nicki Violetti, and then stay a few more days just to enjoy the company of two of my favorite people this side of the universe. The four of us have many connections to many people in this lovely industry of ours, and inevitably, many of those people arose naturally in conversation. What amazed and aggravated me was that the more we talked shop, the more negative we all became, the more bad things we had to say about more people, and the more exasperating it became to simply be involved with any of it.

The overwhelming majority of beef out there is a direct result of trainers, coaches and athletes doing things differently and being convinced that everyone else is doing it wrong. This in and of itself is not necessarily problematic, and is actually exactly what should be happening—if you don't believe what you're doing is the best way to do it, what the fuck are you doing it for? The problem lies in the attitudes that arise within this context, and the public and private belittling of those poor misguided assholes who have yet to learn what each of us knows so well already.

This is not to say that there shouldn't be a running debate among professionals about how to best accomplish any given set of goals—that's how progress is made, along with competition and the resulting comparison of results. However, instead of a civilized and productive exchange of ideas and methods, we get the kind of futile bickering and vicious insults one would expect from children whose parents didn't have the foresight to beat them when appropriate.

This is not remarkably complicated, and I'm not sure why exactly people are having so much trouble not being complete dicks. Maybe it's the internet environment and the sense of safety from repercussion it provides—it's remarkably easy to talk shit when you're not on the receiving end of a fist, and when you're able through cleverness and calculation to create a public persona that conveniently disguises any of your shortcomings. If a hairy 45-year old man in his mother's basement can be a nubile 17 year-old girl online, a mediocre trainer or athlete can pretty easily become elite. Of course, this excuse assumes that we're only polite and friendly in response to the fear of consequences; I'd like to believe that people might be able to simply act with respect for its own sake. Maybe that's a silly notion I should just abandon.

I'm not asking anyone to re-align their chakras, synchronize their vibrational frequencies with each other, hold hands and sing, or any other distasteful new-age tomfoolery; I'd just like to see us focusing on what's important, and what we're ostensibly in business to do—produce better athletes, trainers and coaches.

Josh Everett (no, we're still not related) touched on this in his article last month, *Why Dots*. It takes a lot of time and energy to so vehemently criticize someone or their methods, time and energy that could be much better spent improving your own methods, researching others, experimenting, and training yourself and your athletes. This kind of criticism and juvenile bad-mouthing does nothing to improve your own abilities, and any assistance it provides through ego-stroking is minor and short-lived at best. Further, it limits your ability to contribute to the progress of others by creating a reputation for yourself that most will find repellant. You can take a brash stance and tell these people to go fuck themselves, tell yourself you don't want that kind of lightweight as a client or associate anyway, and return to reveling in your own glory, but it will catch up to you eventually, and when it does, talking yourself out of it with the same tongue that caused the crash will likely not be an option.

If you're convinced that your approach is superior, why not simply continue implementing it, demonstrating its efficacy, and inviting others to learn about it if they so desire? And if they don't—and here's the key—LEAVE THEM THE FUCK ALONE. If their methods are inferior and ineffective, they pose no genuine threat to you or your business, and consequently don't deserve your attention and effort. And when confronted with a challenge, trust in the superiority of your methods to make the case, not personal attacks that have no bearing on the argument at hand.

This really isn't asking that much: Just that professionals be professional.

ASK GREG

Ask Greg is a regular feature we introduced to the Performance Menu in January 2011 in which readers can email their questions for a chance to be answered in the journal. The following are questions from issues 72—86.

Brian Asks: Wouldn't the Jerk Dip Squat be more effective as an explosive exercise? I read a russian book that outlined an exercise of jumping with 50% bodyweight (similar to a "jerk drive" I guess) and it found that those who could jump higher had a higher jerk, even if others had a stronger squat.

Greg Says: More effective for what? To improve the drive of the jerk, yes. But that's not the purpose of the exercise; a jerk dip squat is to develop strength and position. With an athlete who has an inconsistent or improper dip position/movement, adding speed to it just reinforces the problem rather than helping to correct it. In this case, my goal is to practice and strengthen correct positioning, not improve explosiveness.

Jerk drives are great in theory, but I've never seen anyone be able to perform them without pushing the bar forward considerably. This is not a habit I want to encourage. It's also pretty rough on the body to bring the weight back down. You can do them on jerk blocks, but there is the same problem - people will push the bar forward or jump their bodies backward every time; if you try to just drop out from under the bar as it comes back down, you're going to chin check yourself. So then people, consciously or not, cut the drive short to prevent killing themselves, and then they're just training that - not finishing the drive of their jerks.

The best option in my opinion is to do a jumping quarter squat from top or bottom depending on what exactly you want to work on. Bar on traps like a back squat. In a power rack or on jerk blocks. I believe there is a video of this on the site under "jumping squat". If you're working on the jerk specifically, set the start position with an upright torso and knees forward rather than more of a squat position. These can be done light to extremely heavy and there are no problems preventing correct execution at any weight.

Regarding the book, that those athletes who had higher jumps were better jerkers doesn't mean the exercise was responsible; the exercise was, just like the jerk, an opportunity to demonstrate that particular athletic quality. Not to say that it couldn't help, but it's easy to attribute success to things like that when they're not necessarily responsible.

Cheryl Asks: First off thank you for all that you do in the strength and conditioning, fitness, weightlifting and CrossFit worlds; it is very much appreciated. My question is regarding weight-lifting belts—do you need them, if so when? Pros/ cons, proper fit? What type/ brand would you recommend? I've read a lot of information both for and against their use, but I am curious to hear your thoughts on the subject.

Greg Says: Whether or not you need a belt, or should use one, is dependent on who "you" are. The first thing to keep in mind is that in few sports or activities will you be wearing a belt; weightlifting, powerlifting, strongman and throwing are the only ones that come to mind. If training for one of these sports, it makes sense that a belt will have some kind of utility. For an athlete whose sports involves strength and power but is not in a controlled environment that allows a belt, such as a football player, any strength they have will have to be applied without the use of a belt in the game, so it makes sense that these athletes will need to have the trunk strength to support their leg and hip strength. Of course, it's argued sometimes that wearing a belt in training allows the use of more weight, which develops more strength. My opinion is that this doesn't make much sense—if the rest of your body can't support a given degree of strength, you won't be able to use it (at least safely) anyway.

For the abovementioned athletes who can use belts in competition, whether or not to use them is still a choice. I see no reason for a powerlifter to not use a belt. The sport encourages the use of gear, the goal is to move as much weight as possible, and a belt certainly helps that, and I don't see any detriment in wearing one. The same goes for strongman competition—these guys are moving enormous weights, but more importantly, they're putting themselves in compromised positions, and many events have a considerable stamina component. The back tends to give out before the muscles it's supporting, so a belt can be the difference between success or failure and safety or injury. I haven't seen many throwers wear belts, and I'm not sure I think it would be particularly helpful; it strikes me as being more disruptive to fluid movement. That would be a very individual decision.

For the weightlifter, belts are also a pretty individual choice. There's no question that a belt will help a lifter lift more, at least in the clean & jerk. Some find it helpful for maintaining trunk rigidity in the snatch as well, but I find it too cumbersome and prohibitive of proper movement and positioning.

I discourage the use of belts with anything less than 85-90% or so in the squat, clean and jerk. It's important to continuously improve trunk strength along with the rest of the body. When it's time to go big, the addition of a belt will add a bit more on top. Using a belt more frequently and with lighter weights just makes a lifter dependent on it; in some cases, psychologically more than physically.

For weightlifting I prefer nylon belts with cam buckles over leather belts with traditional buckles simply because they're more adjustable and less restrictive. As far as fit goes, the belt should be snugged up a bit tighter than you unbelted brace position—don't crank it down like a corset and turn your trunk into a skinny base that won't support any weight.

Mike Asks: Greg, Aimee, I've got a question. What's the difference, if any, when conducting strength training and the sets and rep scheme is either 5 sets of 3 reps or 3 sets of 5 reps. Conditions: the lifter is new (linear progression/novice) and performing sets across, the total reps would be the same in either scheme, the only difference is the set volume.

Understanding that novice lifters will more than likely not have a true 1rm, but I'd think you'd want to get them as close as possible each session to their 1rm for that day, but still creating reps/vol. So my thought is to put them in a 5 sets of 3 reps scheme with the intent of creating less intensity per set and a little more volume for the session. Examples:

1) Back Squat 3 sets X 5reps @ 100# (total set vol. 500#, total vol. 1500#); or 2) Back Squat 5 sets X 3 reps @ 105# (total set vol. 315#, total vol. 1575#)

I could be totally off here, either way I'd still appreciate your thoughts or observations, especially if this can be applied to o-lifting programming.

Greg Says: The basic difference for anyone will be that 5 sets of 3 reps will allow heavier weights to be used with the same volume—5-10% or so—although that doesn't necessarily mean it needs to be heavier.

With a novice lifter, just about anything works, and especially with young lifters, higher reps often work better. With a new lifter who is still a bit dodgy with his or her movement, staying with somewhat lighter weights is a good idea, so more reps can be used to get enough work in to actually get a training effect.

Max numbers for new lifters are not important, and they're changing so dramatically and frequently, they would be of little use if you had them anyway. That early stage of training is really the time to be more intuitive and make decisions on how the lifter is feeling day to day rather than attempting to devise some clever plan and stick to it. For example, the program I use when new lifters come to Catalyst has no weight prescriptions; just exercises, sets and reps, and even those are flexible. Obviously I have an idea of what I want the athlete to be doing in terms of effort level, but there's really no way of predicting what weights will be necessary, possible and effective, especially in the classic lifts, and I definitely have to change the volume for some people to minimize or prevent joint pain, etc. while they're adapting to the training.

Regarding getting the lifter close to his/her 1RM each session, not really. Depending on how the athlete is conditioned, you may be doing 5 sets of 3 with anywhere from 75-90% of 1RM (and more is totally possible with certain training). If you mean getting them as close to a maximal effort for each set, or for the total sets, then that's more likely, but also not necessarily true. It's usually a good idea to start any cycle/program well within the lifter's present abilities so there's space to gain momentum. For example, if a lifter could grind out 5x3 with 85% on day one of the program, it might be smart to start him at 75-80% and take 2-4 weeks to build up to and then move past that level.

It also depends largely on what other training is accompanying the squatting. If your focus during a given cycle or time in the cycle is heavy classic lifts, or maybe heavy pulling, you won't be able to squat the athlete as heavy, or more likely, with as much volume. In that case, you may be doing 5 sets of 3 with a weight that would otherwise be more appropriate for 5x5.

Tony Asks: Is there going to be an alternative to Crossfit? Perhaps a confederation of gyms that employ similar methods but reject the unscientific basis, random workouts, and ridiculous claims of the Glassman cult? Thank you for your time.

Greg Says: Tough question to answer for a number of reasons. First, I want to clarify that I love the CF community in general and the majority of the people within it; it has put me in touch with a lot of great people, and it's driving exposure to weightlifting, which undeniably helps support my business. That being said, I obviously have significant objections to many of the current philosophies, actions and attitudes of the organization's leadership and those affiliates and individuals who subscribe, support and/or endorse those things. Fortunately I'm better now at not allowing them to interfere with my day to day operations and mood.

I think there already exist informal networks of gyms, coaches and trainers who share similar philosophies and methods. It would be great to have something more organized for the sake of individuals finding coaches and gyms of which they could expect certain levels of professionalism, experience and ability. The problem as I see it is that there is so much variation among such gyms that it would be difficult if not impossible to establish criteria or standards that would be of any utility. Add to that the fact that small, independent gyms are just that: independent. Few if any would want to be obligated to follow any kind of rules, adhere to any kind of plan, etc that originated outside of their own business. And if the confederation is loose enough to prevent those kinds of objections, I don't see it being very useful.

James Fitzgerald is doing about as close to what you're describing that I know of with his coaching certification and affiliation and associate coach system. A good indicator of the program's quality is the following question and answer from the certification page:

Q: I've been coaching a long time, can I bypass one of the levels?

A: No.

The CrossFit concept will eventually be ubiquitous like Pilates or yoga with complete decentralization, and at that point it will be possible for someone else to step in and reorganize those individuals who are most serious about training into a more refined, focused and professional system than exists now.

Rich Asks: I've been doing crossfit for about 18 months and train 5 times per week. I would like to dial in some supplemental lifting in order to build strength. I've heard that the deadlift is a great all body exercise (it benefits all parts of the body with strength gains) and I would like to build my shoulder strength. What programming would you recommend to work in with crossfit with my 5 day workout (Thursday and Sunday off) if I want to add deadlifts and shoulder strength? Thanks for you help!

Greg Says: First, building strength is obviously your primary goal right now, so the most important thing is to treat it accordingly. In my opinion, that means completely changing your perspective—don't work in some strength training with your CrossFit; work in some CrossFit with your strength training. This is how people end up spinning their wheels for so long—they never actually put real focus on what they say their goals are because they're worried about slipping in some other area (classic CF problem). Your conditioning doesn't have to suffer much, and it will come back very quickly.

There's no one program I would recommend for this—just about anything you do will increase your strength coming out of a strict CF program. The deadlift is great, but I would spend more time on the squat, which will make your deadlift go up as well. For pressing strength, focus on the press and push press.

Here's a very simple example:

Monday: Back squat
Wednesday: Press
Thursday: Deadlift

Week 1: 60% x 8 x 4 (DL 2 sets)
Week 2: 75% x 5 x 5 (DL 3 sets)
Week 3: 80% x 4 x 4 (DL 2 sets)
Week 4: 85% x 3 x 3 (DL 1 set)
Week 5: 90% x 1 x 3 (DL 1 set)
Week 6: Test Max
(weight x reps x sets)

If you don't know your maxes for any of these, follow the same set/rep prescriptions and feel out appropriate weights for each.

This is a minimalist strength program and it assumes you'll be doing a lot of other work (i.e. CrossFit) along with it, and doing a lot of squatting, pulling, pressing variants at a range of repetitions and weights.

You can also just dig around for canned strength programs (e.g. the popular short list 5/3/1, Bill Starr's 5x5 stuff, etc) and then work your CrossFit around those. Take it easy on leg-related conditioning work or you'll quickly find yourself in a hole.

Becky Asks: I've been Crossfitting for about 2 years, but in the last 5 months I've been trying to improve my Olympic lifts. What are some good exercises to help me get under the bar faster? I have flexibility issues, so my squat isn't perfect, which adds to the problem. But I'm just not fast enough yet. Thanks so much for your help!

Greg Says: Your movement under the bar can be slow for a few different reasons, and that will affect what exercises help. If it's truly the pull under the bar that's slow, it may be a strength issue, a technique issue, or a lack of aggressiveness. I'm going to discuss everything using the snatch, but you'll be able to apply it to the clean pretty easily.

Let's worry about strength first. You can think of the third pull in three basic parts: the initial pull of the body down toward the bar, the turnover of the bar, and the punch up under the bar. Each of these parts can be strengthened best individually because one usually limits the weights than can be used for others, but can also be trained together with certain exercises.

For the initial pull under, it's an issue of arm, back and shoulder strength—the ability to forcefully pull the elbows up and out. The simplest exercise to strengthen this movement would be a tall snatch high-pull. You won't be able to use a lot of weight—it's not a strong movement for anyone—but this is pure upper body strength in exactly the position and movement you want. You may not even be able to use an empty barbell—you may need to use a lighter technique bar or even dumbbells. Stick with 5-6 reps, 3-5 sets.

You can also do snatch high-pulls from the mid- or upper-thigh and use the legs and hips to accelerate the bar initially, then use the upper body to finalize the pull to the top position. This will allow you to use more weight as well as better simulate an actual lift. Stay flat-footed if you want to emphasize the upper body more, as this will force you to limit how much hip and leg speed you can put on the bar.

To use even more weight, do snatch high-pulls from the floor with maximal speed.

To strengthen the turnover of the bar, you'll need to use some muscle snatch or long pull variation. You can use the same kind of principles described above for the high-pull. To completely isolate the upper body movement, perform a muscle snatch from the tall position, which means you get no leg or hip at all. These will be very light—don't make the mistake of trying to load it up or you'll end up changing the movement, which defeats the purpose. You can add more weight by doing the muscle snatch from the hang or floor. Snatch long pulls are another good exercise for turnover strength because they keep more tension on the upper body throughout the movement.

Finally, to strengthen the punch up under the bar, use snatch balances or drop snatches. Drop snatches will not allow you to use as much weight, so if you want to load it up, do a snatch balance. These are also great exercises to improve your speed and timing in the very last portion of the third pull (which is really a push).

Strength may not be the problem; it may be technique. If you're not moving yourself and the bar optimally, your pull under will be slower than it should be. Be sure your elbows are rotated to point to the sides throughout the first and second pulls so they will remain properly oriented upon entrance into the third pull. Don't worry about shrugging under the bar—pull with your arms and the shrug will come along at the right time and to the right degree. Pull the elbows up and out and keep your body and the bar in immediate proximity—the bar should be close enough to smell on your way past it.

Continue pulling the elbows up even as your turn the arms over—keep tension on throughout the movement. It's common to see lifters suddenly get slack in the system at this point, and that only slows them down and increases the chance of an unstable receipt of the bar. As you finish the turnover, flip the hands back into the proper position and punch up under the bar with a relatively loose grip. This entire movement must be fluid and extremely aggressive.

You can use tall snatches to work on the entire movement. Focus on keeping your weight back over the feet rather than shifting forward as you initiate the movement. Have someone stand at your side and make sure you're keeping the bar and your body as close to each other as possible.

This leads to the final consideration: that your lack of speed under the bar is actually coming from earlier in the lift. Many athletes are so focused on the upward extension of the pull that they continue pulling long after it's productive. You have an extremely brief moment when the bar is weightless at the apex of its elevation, and if you're not already moving under the bar, you're losing the opportunity. The moment your hips and knees reach their final extended position, you must transition your feet and pull under—the finish and initiation of the pull under should really occur almost simultaneously rather than one after the other. In order for this to happen, it's critical that the bar and the hips meet properly—the snap of the hips into extension will actually help get them back and moving into the squatting position faster.

To work on this, you can high-hang snatches or power snatches—this will allow you to better focus on the final extension and change of direction. You can also snatch or power snatch off of high blocks (mid-thigh or higher).

Finally, focus on being aggressive throughout the entire lift, every time you lift. You have to develop that mindset every time you train.

Mike Asks: I have been swinging kettlebells for about forty years. I have old Milo kettlebells that were at least forty years old back when I started. I have a pretty good collection of old books, magazines and "courses" going back more than 100 years. Until the recent "Russian" kettlebell training rebirth I was never aware of anyone swinging one kettlebell with two hands. I have never seen a kettlebell with a handle made to fit two hands.

Swinging a pair of kettlebells outside the knees (as one would swing a pair of Clubbells) allows one to keep the back "flat" and the shoulders back/tight allowing for a better focus in the hip snap in the swing. If someone has short arms and/or a long torso it is nearly impossible to hold one kettlebell with two hands swinging it beneath the crotch while maintaining proper back and shoulder position. Where did this two-hands on one kettlebell come from? And, why?

In the old days the dumbbell swing was a popular exercise, but it was done with one hand, and the dumbbell was swung to an overhead, locked-out position. I have seen a photo of a swing done with a short barbell or long dumbbell with two hands, but it was never prescribed this way as an exercise that I am aware of.

Greg Says: Great question. Short answer: No idea; I'm not much of a historian. I would assume the two-handed swing was popularized because it's easier to do "safely" than a one-arm swing, and particularly a one-arm swing outside the legs. While it may be a bit crowded for bigger guys, you have no lateral rotational force to contend with, so you have less concern for people getting squirrely and hurting their delicate little backs. The Strength & Health era is much different than the RKC era—back then, the people who wanted to train wanted to train, and they weren't poised to hire a lawyer to sue over a back injury.

With a one-handed swing outside the legs, there is also the potential for careless or uncoordinated people to wrecking-ball their own knee—also not recommended. Finally, with this kind of swing, it behooves one to use a narrower stance to avoid said wrecking-ball action, and most people have more trouble setting a solid back arch with a narrower stance.

Maybe the above is a fairly cynical interpretation. It may just be that over time the exercise naturally evolved into what it is today based on people's experiences training, and the two-hands swing was viewed as a bit more useful or effective. I like the two-hands swing, but I also really like the one-hand swing between the legs—great trunk and hip stability exercise.

Erik Asks: As someone who primarily Olympic lifts, what are the most proactive and/or least detrimental things I can do if I want to "workout" when I can't get to a gym for up to a week?

Greg Says: That's a tough one. Unfortunately there is really no way to train optimally for weightlifting without a barbell. But it's not completely hopeless. I would spend time on explosive bodyweight exercises, particularly jumping exercises, and core work.

Tuck jumps, bounding, broad jumps, and squat jumps are all good exercises that will keep you firing quickly when you're not training. Obviously there are an endless number of ab exercises you can do without equipment, and you can figure out some back exercises without equipment, even if it's just doing supermans on the floor; also try hyperextensions or reverse hypers on a variety of furniture or similar.

General bodyweight exercises like squats, lunges and push-ups won't hurt either. They'll be good for maintaining mobility and keeping you moving; just don't turn it into a bootcamp session. I would keep rep numbers to 10-15 at the most and don't rush through sets or exercises.

Jake Asks: I have a horrendously weak trunk/back stemming from ignorance in training and a couple fractured vertebrae (L4/L5) in high school (I'm 26). I found the "Back Training for Weightlifting" article and am starting it tomorrow with the only limitation being lack of access to reverse hyperextensions. What would be a good substitute for these and do you have any suggestions for a similar work out program for the rest of the trunk (obliques, abs, etc)? I'm not going for a six-pack, but like I said I've just recently gotten into lifting and know this is a weak area that is limiting my lifts and increasing my likelihood for injury, which I seem to have a tendency for already.

Greg Says: Reverse hypers can be done on a number of things such as tables—you may not be able to drop your legs to a completely vertical bottom position, but it's better than nothing.

With ab training, I like a lot of variety. Each training day, pick an exercise for static holds, trunk flexion, lateral trunk flexion or trunk rotation as your primary exercise. Do 3-5 sets, and vary resistance and rep-range: 8-10 reps with weighted exercises, and 20-30 or so with unweighted exercises. Then if you want to throw in another exercise on a given day, pick another movement type (I would recommend doing some kind of plank variation if your primary movement was dynamic).

In your case, the focus should be preventing any compromise of normal spinal range of motion and position. That is, avoiding hyperextension, extreme flexion, and extreme rotation. Work only in a range of motion that is 100% pain-free and doesn't cause pain afterward. I would make plank variations a big emphasis, but you MUST ensure that you're holding a proper position. Work in small bursts of 8-10 seconds initially with perfect positions and build up to longer holds or add weight for more short holds. Never progress by allowing a compromise in posture.

Mike Asks: Please consider a Newsletter or other forum for discussing the rationale and recov-

ery implications for training multiple days in a row. I know those in the Oly community take it for granted that a 3 or 4 on, 1 off schedule is standard, but to those of us new to the sport it is less obvious why this is so different from any other form of weight training in terms of ability to do this productively over time. As someone who has trained all his life and has competed in powerlifting, it is not intuitive that training 4 or 5 days in a row is something one can recover from, regardless of age. What is unique about the Olympic lifts that require so much volume; and why can one recover from this more so than any other kind of resistance training? Is it because the eastern Europeans do it? Then again, for those of us living a normal life, not 18 – 22 years old, and drug free, it becomes much harder to adapt to this. I have found the Oly lifts much more taxing than any powerlifting training I ever did, due no doubt to the nervous system load from high power output and concentration on form. No such thing as "walking through" a Greg Everett workout! It would also seem that your workouts run counter to the recommendations of your friend Robb Wolf, who is so acutely concerned about cortisol and overtraining.

As a side note, I get regular blood work from a sports medicine doctor. She recently informed me that my cortisol levels are through the roof, and said it is clearly from overtraining. While I am 52 and know that is a big part of it, I still question whether anyone with a real job/life can handle the rigors of daily high output training. Please comment.

Greg Says: Very interesting topic, and I will try to do it justice. First, I wouldn't say that weightlifting *requires* high-volume and frequency training, but certainly it's a common approach. It's also important to acknowledge that volume and frequency are relative, and what's high to one athlete may be moderate or even low for another. Within my own gym I have some lifters who thrive on 400-500 reps per week, while others can handle only 200 or fewer, and this doesn't always align with age.

The snatch, clean and jerk are more complex than the powerlifting squat, bench and deadlift by orders of magnitude; the degrees of technical skill involved in the two pursuits are not even comparable. I don't say this to disparage powerlifting or powerlifters in any way, but it's an unavoidable truth, and it plays a role in training differences. This being the case, it's obvious that in order to master the competitive lifts, far more time and far more quality reps must be performed by the weightlifter than the powerlifter. Weightlifting is a unique sport in that the lifts inextricably link the motor qualities of precise movement and timing with strength and speed. Powerlifting has a huge strength component, but minimal skill; something like pitching a baseball has a huge skill component, but minimal strength. People are not usually resistant to the idea of a baseball pitcher throwing a lot of balls in a day, week, month or year, because the need to practice the skill is obvious. The skill of weightlifting is not as obvious because most people are viewing it from a perspective largely shaped by history with bodybuilding and powerlifting training.

Next, there is an issue of adaptation. Anything you do that is a sudden and significant increase in volume, intensity or frequency is going to hurt. The key is that elite weightlifters didn't begin training 6 days a week with 600 reps; the best of the best spend years developing in well-designed programs that allowed them to build the conditioning for this volume of work. Do drugs play a role in many cases? It's inarguable that drug use will allow you to train heavier with more volume and frequency, but being drug free does not mean you can't adapt to high volume and frequency (just not as high and not as quickly). You're able to walk every day without a problem. That's leg training seven days a week; but you're adapted to that particular intensity and volume level. The same thing can be accomplished with lifting to a great extent.

The snatch and clean & jerk are less systemically taxing than squats and deadlifts because they're smaller percentages of a true total body maximal effort, although in many cases, not that much smaller. This alone means they can be done more frequently by anyone. The classic lifts also overwhelmingly train neurological adaptations rather than morphological ones, which also means you're not waiting around for tissue remodeling between workouts ala the bodybuilder.

Also, complete recovery between training sessions is not something that the weightlifter is necessary striving for; instead, you're looking at blocks of training sessions to create a cumulative effect.

Training multiple consecutive days also doesn't mean that every day is maximal intensity and volume. Day to day volume and intensity will fluctuate to allow some degree of restoration. Even Bulgarian-style purists use such modulation— they just allow the body to dictate the timing and degree rather than planning for it ahead of time.

Having spent most of your training life with an infrequent schedule means you're conditioned, physically and psychologically, to just that. With time and a smart progression, there is no reason you wouldn't be able to significantly increase your training volume and frequency. Of course, being 52 with real life obligations and the attendant stress will ultimately limit what you can do. But again, it's all relative. You just need to experiment to find what works best for you, but build up to those experiments wisely.

Regarding cortisol levels, I'm not sure how your doctor can be certain high levels are due to overtraining; stress is stress, whether it comes from training, work, family complications, poor sleep, etc. Any given level of training could be "overtraining" if the rest of the stress in your life exceeds a tolerable threshold. So in such a case, why is it overtraining, and not overworking, under-sleeping, over-having-your-wife-use-your-credit-card?

Derek Asks: I recently injured my back and now that I am starting to lift again I can still feel it when weights start approaching heavy as well as mentally. Today I did a 7x3 of real light 1 1/4 quarter squats with a 1 second pause on initial squat. The whole session felt really great and beneficial for form and strenghtening up my weak points. I was wondering if continuing a linear progression of 1 1/4 squats starting real light has any merit while my back heals up and I get more comfortable again. Thanks.

Greg Says: Absolutely. There's really no way to plan the recovery timeline for an injury—you'll make quick progress at times and other times you'll regress somewhat. Whatever you're doing to come back from that injury will need to be flexible to accommodate this. Starting light and comfortable and building up gradually is a smart way to go, but there may be times when you need to back off a bit.

Squatting at a more controlled speed will help ensure you're maintaining your positions, limit the chance to re-injure your back, and give the spinal stabilizers more time under tension to develop the isometric strength necessary to maintain posture. Make trunk stability a focus during the squats and take this opportunity to perfect the position and movement so that when you're healthy, you will have actually improved technically, not just returned to previous function.

Dan Asks: Hi! Love the performance menu and look forward to reading it each month. I am originally a crossfitter that have obtained certs and stuff, and am a student of your Oly class held in Chico a couple of years ago. Anyway the reason I'm writing is being a "trainer" for the past three years it has become obvious that there is a difference of someone who holds a cert and one that is actually a trainer.

I am 40 year old, Fire Captain and Part Owner of a recently opened crossfit gym. That being said what would you suggest outside of attending college again, of increasing my education in a systematic way as a trainer? I do not want to be a trainer that just has a one size fits all approach, but I feel I need education in the following areas: Body Types and how to approach training; Clueing in on injury prone motions (have seemed to hurt a lot of my clients when I first started, way too many pull ups); Helping clients state observable and obtainable goals.

If you could address this for a trainer that does have time to go back to school but is passionate about seeing their clients progress uninjured, and obtaining measurable goals.

Greg Says: Definitely don't go back to college. The best way to learn more about these things is to interact with other more experienced trainers and coaches to find out what they do. These are the guys who often have the classroom education, but have since spent years in the gym experimenting and finding out what actually works and what doesn't. Sometimes theory falls apart completely in practice, and sometimes it holds up well. You won't know until you implement it. Some coaches and gyms offer internships or mentorship programs, some less formal than others—this would be ideal. But since you're not a kid fresh out of college with no job or responsibilities, this is likely not a practical option for you. However, I would still contact local coaches you respect and see if they'd be willing to let you shadow them occasionally, or even set up private sessions for you to ask questions and discuss various practices rather than actually train—I've done this quite a few times and if other coaches have the time, many are open to doing the same as long as they don't feel you're a competitor.

The internet also offers a ridiculous amount of help in this area. Particularly

THE PORTABLE GREG EVERETT

with the current trend of posting just about everything you do online, you can find out what many coaches and programs are doing without having to actually be there. Granted, most smarter coaches won't disclose everything, but you can still get a lot of good ideas.

Try setting aside a certain amount of time each week for continuing education—whether that's reading new books, websites or speaking with other trainers.

Shane Asks: I don't know if there is even an answer to this question. I just started running a dedicated oly lift class once a week at our box. Membership and time constraints just don't allow me to run a class any more often than that. I feel completely confident and in my element running a class for either beginners or for intermediate/more advanced athletes. The situation is that I will have both showing up to the same class. Can you give me any advice on how to run a class where some people have no business lifting more than PVC or an unloaded barbell, yet others should be working with full training loads and doing more advanced weighted skills and drills? I'm thinking the only answer is to run separate classes, but I would really appreciate your feedback and advice if you feel there is another way to go. Thanks! Hope to see you in June at your seminar!

Greg Says: This is a tough situation, but one that you'll always have to deal with. In a given training session at Catalyst, I may have a couple national championship level lifters, some lifters not at national level yet, and a lifter who can barely overhead squat below parallel.

In your situation, you'll need to prioritize your attention to those who need it most, i.e. the least experienced lifters. For the more advanced lifters, you should be able to write a program that keeps them busy and working independently while you actually coach the newer athletes. During this time, obviously you'll need to actually interact with the more advanced lifters, but this can be done concisely because they should know what you're talking about when you give them a cue.

I would suggest having a plan for maybe three levels of experience each day you come in—if someone at one of those levels shows up, you know what you're doing; if they don't, it doesn't matter. The hardest way to do it is to come up with a plan on the fly based on who happens to show up to class. The advanced guys may be on a long-term program, while with the beginners you may just choose a series of drills to work on in each session. But if you actually have a plan going into it, you can get everyone started and keep them moving. This also frees you up a bit to adjust what the beginners are doing since they'll probably need some flexibility built into their training.

Anonymous Asks: I know you probably have a lot to do so I'll make this quick. I'm new to Olympic lifting. I'm 26 yrs old 6' 205lbs, powerlifting background (best raw lifts BP-455

DL-585 BS-605 at a bodyweight of 265). I just recently got into CrossFit and lost 55 lbs using paleo + CrossFit two times a week. I fell in love with the Olympic lifts. So far I can Power Clean and Power Snatch more than I can regular clean and snatch. Flexibility issues are getting better but mechanics are taking some time. Currently I have power snatched 225 lbs and power clean and jerked 315 lbs. I want to compete!!! However I have very little coaching or access to equipment.

Question—or questions—I used a lot speed training in the past for powerlifting and it worked really well for me. So I was wondering if throwing in some 50-60% doubles or triples (focused on bar speed) for maybe 5 to 8 sets would help the same way in Olympic lifts as well as powerlifting? Also, I'm using all the resources I have (mostly your site, Mike Burgener, and youtube) to find training info with what little time and money I have to improve my knowledge and ability in Olympic lifting. I just have zero access to anyone (coaches or athletes) of elite or even competitive status. I really feel as though I can be competitive at 94 kg in this sport. I guess your could say I'm throwing a penny in the email wishing well. What can I do?

P.S. I live in the north Georgia mountains (very isolated). Just so you know the closest Olympic lifting team I can find is in savannah GA more 8 hours away.

Greg Says: First, decide how important lifting is to you, and if it's really important, move to a place with a team you want to train with. At 26, you might not have too many obligations or ties yet and this may still be possible. Do it while you can if that's what you want. Nothing will help you improve more or at a faster rate than working with a good coach and training with a team of dedicated lifters.

Regarding lifts at 50-60% with a speed focus, yes, I like this a lot. Generally I wouldn't go as light as 50% with the actual competition lifts—60% would be a bottom end—but I might on things like high or mid-hang, high block work, or combinations of power and squat lifts (50-60% would be of the squat variation). This is a really good way of getting a large volume of mechanically sound and quick lifts in, and it can be done without being very taxing, so you're still able to do the heavy work you need.

For someone with a good strength base like you have, but at the moment limited flexibility and technique, this should be very helpful. Being strong, it can be easy to work with weights heavier than you should be and constantly be stuck lifting in a technically unsound manner, which just reinforces the problems you're trying to correct. Build your lift-specific strength with pulling variations, squats and pressing variations while you develop your technical ability and speed, and as the latter elements improve, you'll be able to move into training the classic lifts heavier more regularly.

Carl Asks: I really appreciate the Ask Greg section of the magazine, as it seems every question you've answered is one I wanted to ask. Greg, thanks for the straightforward strength approach for CrossFitters that you outlined in the March issue. I have researched some of the canned programs and they all recommend doing supplemental exercises (dips, wtd pullups, etc) regularly, as well. Do you have a strong opinion about their value?

I really benefited by Scotty's article on higher carb paleo, especially the simple but effective ways of checking your body's reaction to the paleo diet. I immediately went out to get a thermometer to test my thyroid function!

Can you tell me if he has covered dietary supplements and their timing? I take fish oil and D3 in the morning and the evening (mainly because it is easy to remember to take them with breakfast and dinner), but a friend has suggested that spreading out the doses during the day is better.

Thanks again for your excellent advice. Keep up the great work.

Greg Says: I like supplemental exercises, but you have to be careful about getting carried away with them. Many people try to do everything all the time and suddenly end up with 4-hour training sessions because of all the accessory work they cobble onto the skeleton of their program, or worse, they end up cutting down on the volume of the exercises they should be prioritizing to accommodate the accessory work. There are certain things that need to be included based on what the program consists of and the athlete's needs. For example, I like to almost always include some kind of upper body pulling work for lifters to build and maintain scapular stability and balance out all the pressing and overhead work they do. Pull-ups and rowing variations are the staples. So the value of accessory work will vary quite a bit depending on the athlete, the time, and the rest of the program.

Regarding the fish oil and vitamin D, if you're not taking a huge amount (which you shouldn't be with those two things), breakfast and dinner is fine. Fish oil is best taken with food for better absorption. Vitamin D can also be taken in the evening before bed to help with sleep, although I can't vouch for the effectiveness of this. I would say that dividing the doses between the first and last meals of the day is spreading it out adequately.

Sam Asks: A couple of questions I struggle with regularly. I know for both of these it depends on the day, how you are feeling, etc. but looking for general guidance.

1) How many lifts do you usually take to work up to a "heavy single" Sn or CJ? This would be excluding light warm-ups at say 50% or less. As an example, my current max is 78 and my last heavy single workout looked like this: 40x2, 50x2, 55, 60, 63, 66, 69, 71, 73(f), 73, 75(f), 75, 77, 78. This was a total of 16 lifts including the 2 missed lifts. This feels like it might be too much but I am not sure.

2) Related to above, what sort of jumps (%) do you take in getting to a heavy single, 3-5% is my guess.

Greg Says: How you approach this depends on your goal for the workout, the lift, and what you're conditioned for. If the primary goal is to simply hit the heaviest weight possible, you're technically consistent, and you're used to taking big jumps, then usually we want to move up to the heavy single with as few lifts as possible. However, if you're not technically consistent, this can be a terrible idea. In this case, usually taking smaller jumps as you near your top weight will keep you more consistent and technically sound, which will allow you to finish at a higher weight. If you instead try to make bigger jumps and the lift falls apart, you're expending a lot of energy to miss lifts; even if you try to come back down, you may be mentally defeated at that point and not be able to work back up. 3-5% is a good starting point as you get above 80% or so. Often athletes get concerned about wasting energy taking so many lifts, but if you're not technically developed enough to take big jumps, your lifts won't be that physically taxing anyway, and you'll end up lifting more if you can maintain confidence and technical consistency longer.

Khaled Asks: I am a CrossFit trainer at CrossFit Norwalk, and I am writing to you regarding programming of dedicated Olympic lifting sessions with a regular CrossFit schedule. I know many high-level CrossFitters will do extra oly lifting work in addition to the CrossFit WODs, but having tried to use the Intermediate Program on p291 of The Complete Guide, I found that the 3-on-1-off-2-on program didn't permit enough time for recovery. On the other hand, doing Olympic lifting occasionally whenever it might happen to pop up in the CrossFit variable programming doesn't seem regular enough to produce consistent growth or results.

Do you have any recommendations for programming Olympic Lifting sessions in the context of CrossFit? Is it a good idea to just focus on the classic lifts and leave the other stuff (squats, DLs, core) to the WODs? Or would you suggest taking these latter elements out of the WODs and separating them out? Basically, this would result in no 'pure strength' days in the CrossFit programming (presumably having more rest days, since you'd only have metcons), and having a completely separate schedule for the Olympic lifting/strength development that follows its own progression and rest schedule.

I have been trying to sort this out for a long time, but haven't been able to do so to my satisfaction, which is why I'm e-mailing you. Getting things to sort with CrossFit is only the first step, since I also train as a gymnast 3 times a week. I sincerely want to find a way to be really good at Olympic Lifting, gymnastics, and metabolic work capacity, as much as it is possible. Any help or advice you could provide would be greatly appreciated.

Greg Says: First, you have to understand that all of this training needs to be integrated in some fashion—you'll never get ideal results if you simply try to force two distinct training programs together. In other words, it needs to be a single program that covers all of the aspects you're attempting to train.

In my opinion, a strength program should be the foundation of any Cross-Fit program (I'm including Olympic lifts when I say strength program). As a corollary to this, I believe crossfit.com should not be a part of anyone's program; there is no plan, no progression, and no sense at all.

What I would suggest is prioritizing. Decide what qualities are most important to you and literally order them. For example, if you're a competitive gymnast and that's your primary focus, improvement of gymnastics skills should be at the top of your list. Whatever this primary focus is, the rest of your training should be built around it. Develop a basic training plan for that primary goal, and then move down the list adding training for each element in appropriate quantity given its ranking. Initially, don't worry about doing too much—just get it all down and see what you have. Once you have that basic plan, you'll more than likely need to trim it down to a reasonable volume of training; again, pare it down based on priorities.

The reality is that you can't do everything at once with the same emphasis; if you have multiple broad athletic goals, you'll need to alternate emphases to some degree over time. This doesn't mean you train one thing and neglect everything else; it simply means you set aside more time and energy to what you've determined is most important at that time.

As an example, let's say you're comfortable with your current gymnastics abilities and are more interested in improving your weightlifting at the moment. Consider spending 1-3 months focusing on lifting and reducing the amount of time you spend training gymnastics. You might lift 3 days/week, train gymnastics 2 days instead of your current 3 and throw in 1-3 relatively short conditioning workouts each week, likely after your gymnastics training. After this period of emphasis, you might shift to a gymnastics focus with more conditioning or whatever you then feel takes priority.

Just remember that it takes a lot less training to maintain capacity than develop it; just because you're not training a given quality at 100%, it won't disappear.

David Asks: How can I get more height out of my pull during snatches and cleans? A lot of the time, I feel like I can not pull the bar high enough to get under it, especially in the clean. Are snatch/clean high pulls my best bet, or do you recommend something else? Thanks!

Greg Says: I can't think of a time I've ever seen a relatively new lifter unable to elevate the bar adequately with the exception of occasional errors. It's typical for these individuals to be snatching and cleaning fractions of their basic strength numbers, and their pulling strength usually far exceeds their classic lift numbers. In other words, without seeing you lift, I would venture a guess that the actual height of the bar is not the problem.

If for some reason you genuinely are unable to elevate the bar sufficiently, then pull variations and strength improvement in general is what you need. High-pulls are not intended to get you pulling the bar higher in the snatch and clean—bar height is not achieved by pulling with the arms. They're intended to do things like train proper bar/body proximity and strengthen the third pull. You can do high-pulls in addition to heavier pulls, but understand that you're not trying to high-pull the bar when doing the actual lifts.

Add more pulls to your program and more variations like pulls from high blocks to emphasize the final explosion. You can also try a complex of a pull + lift, eg snatch pull + snatch to both strengthen the pull and also encourage a complete pull when actually lifting. Power snatches and cleans and work from the hang or blocks will also help you develop more force at the top of the pull and consequently more bar height.

If bar height isn't really the problem as I suspect, I would guess the issue is more related to your change of direction after the pull and your pull under the bar not being fast enough. The height of the bar doesn't matter if you can't get under it in time. Hang and block lifts are great for improving this.

Steve Asks: Years ago I understood that in order to increase muscle size/ strength that there was scientific information that instructed us to overload and muscle to failure or almost failure and than to rest that muscle for 40 hours in order to recover. Some new programs have you working the same muscle after only 24 hours. What is the latest info on this training tip?

Greg Says: This sounds like standard bodybuilding protocol, which largely informs the public's understanding of training in general. If bodybuilding is what you're doing, than this is reasonable advice, although there is quite a bit of variation within bodybuilding and certainly more than one approach works.

When we're talking about training in more of an athletic vain, it's rare to train to failure. This is generally considered ineffective and even counterproductive. Whereas with bodybuilding, the basic idea is to create significant damage to the muscle and then allow morphological supercompensation, athletes are interested primarily in qualities like strength, power and speed more than hypertrophy. When hypertrophy is a goal, more bodybuilding-esque training is often included, and this may involve exercises done to failure or nearly so with less frequency, so this doesn't really deviate from what you're talking about.

The rest of the training will still remain focused on athletic qualities. You're able to walk every day, which is a leg exercise, without detriment. Why? Because it's such a common, frequently performed "exercise" that your body is entirely accommodated to it and it has virtually no effect anymore. This same thing can and does happen with any other exercise to some extent. If an athlete squats the same weight with the same volume every day, eventually (surprisingly quickly, in fact), it will cease to cause soreness or even much fatigue. When you're training in a way that involves many similar movements frequently, you develop not only this foundation of accommodation, but the ability to recover more rapidly (again, this isn't taking the same exercise to failure every day, and certainly not with heavy full-body lifts).

So if you look at a week for a weightlifter, for example, nearly invariably he or she will squat every day in one way or another; this may be actually doing front or back squats every day, or it will be a combination of exercises that involve a squat such as squats, cleans, snatches, etc. These are all "leg exercises", but aside from the athlete having the ability to manage frequent training and recover more quickly than an untrained individual (or one used to training by the protocol you describe), the exercises vary in a number of ways, from the actual movement to the loading to the reps to the total volume. It's this modulation that helps makes it possible to train like this.

In short, I don't know that there's really any "new" information on this; just different groups of people training different ways that have different effects and consequently different protocols.

Steve Asks: Greg, I have been following CrossFit for about 18 months and seen great results. James Fitzgerald is now my coach and I'm trying to really up my game. I have one issue though…. Front Rack position. Do you two have any good suggestions/exercises for me to increase flexibility in this area? Wrist, elbow, shoulder? Also, any movements to increase elbow speed when getting under the bar in the clean. Thanks for your time. Love the blog, it is a tremendous resource.

Greg Says: First, play with your hand spacing on the bar and find the position that gets you the closest with your current flexibility. Often this is wider than you feel like you should be gripping. I generally prefer a wider clean grip for a number of reasons, such as a quicker turnover and better positioning during the pull under, but a wider grip also often makes the rack position easier for people.

Improving flexibility for the rack position is fairly straightforward, but like any other flexibility limitations, it requires consistency and patience. As a start, front squat a lot and consider the exercise a stretch. Emphasize pushing the shoulders forward and up, the elbows up and the palms up above the fingers.

Wrist flexibility is pretty simple: Find ways to push you hand back and hold it. Probably the easiest way to do this is to press your palm against a wall with your arm perpendicular to the wall. Do this both with the fingers pointing up and down. As you loosen up, you can move your arm past perpendicular to close the angle between the hand and forearm further. You can also do this stretch against the floor while in a squat position to combine the two stretches/warm-ups and save time. All the grip work in lifting can make for very tight wrist and finger flexors, so stretch them frequently throughout the day.

The elbows really shouldn't be stretched per se—they primarily just need to become conditioned to the stress of lifting. Spend time warming them up before training by doing elbow circles both directions while rotating your hand to get the ulna and radius moving as much as possible at the elbow. You can also place a bar on your back as you would for a back squat with your hands close to you shoulders, then lift your elbows high in front of you. Gradually move your grip wider as you loose up.

Being able to move your shoulder blades well is important to get the shoulders up and under the bar properly. A combination of scap push-ups and scap ring rows is a good place to start. For the push-up, from a standard push-up position, with an emphasis on a straight, rigid body and the head in line with the back, keep the elbows locked and let your torso sink down by allowing the shoulder blades to retract completely. From that bottom position, push the shoulders forward as far as possible (scapular protraction). Hold each position for a second before changing directions. The ring rows are the identical movement, but with resistance against scapular retraction rather than protraction. You can alternate the two exercises for 3-4 sets of 10-15.

Finally, you can try loading up a bar in a squat rack a bit lower than what you would use to actually squat from. Get your hands on the bar in the position you would grip for a front squat, walk yourself under the bar in a partial squat position, and pushing your shoulders forward and up and your elbows as high as possible, squat yourself up into the bar. If you have a partner, he or she can assist and lift your elbows further than you can do on your own.

As far as elbow speed goes in the clean, check out the article Improving the Clean through a Better Turnover.

Anonymous Asks: I am trying to learn a new skill that is giving me all sorts of problems. Over the last few months I have been working on increasing my shoulder range of motion so that I can get my arms "back" into a good overhead position. At the same time I have been working hard on my front squat. Not so much in trying to lift heavy, but to groove the movement down so I don't fall forward at the bottom.

I thought I had made progress in both areas until I tried something real simple... Get into a bottom squat position and try to press up some light kettlebells. In the bottom position I could barely get my arms overhead. My arms come forward and I feel "stuck" mid range. It almost feels like my scapulae don't want to rotate. With this lack of ROM and stability, there is no way I will ever be able to load beyond PVC pipe.

How often do you see this with new lifters? What drills can I start doing to get past this?

I am patient, and will spend the extra time to get beyond this. I spent a year retooling my dead lift so I would no longer trash my back, and this is next on my list. Thanks for any help you can offer.

Greg Says: Trying to press KBs from the bottom of a squat is not necessarily a good measure of your overhead squat progress. With the arms independent, you have to press straight up, which means the shoulders are being asked to open more than they would need to in a typical wide-grip barbell overhead squat. So if you're still working on that wide-grip overhead squat position, a 2-arm KB or DB overhead squat or Sots press is well beyond what you should expect to be able to do at present.

I'm a proponent of the shotgun approach to flexibility cases like this where

I can't see what exactly is happening—do every stretch you can think of as much as possible. As you progress, you'll feel which ones seem to help and you can start dropping the ones that aren't contributing as much. Definitely spend time on scapular mobility and stability (mainly strengthening your ability to retract and depress the scapulae). Some good exercises for this are band pull-downs, ring rows done properly, and scapular depression/retraction while hanging from a pull-up bar (use a fairly wide grip).

Don't forget to consider upper back, hip and ankle flexibility—if you feel you have good ROM and stability when standing, but lose it when squatting, at least some of it is coming out of your hips and ankles. If you can't sit into a proper upright squat, you can't expect to achieve a sound overhead position for the Olympic lifts.

Anonymous Asks: Greg or Aimee, I was wondering if you could speak to how the feel of the classical lifts seems to change as the bar weight approaches and goes beyond body weight, as I just found out today while cleaning. Here's what I mean. I am a powerlifter who is trying to transition into Oly lifting, so my base of strength is good. When it comes to cleaning I have found that I can power clean more than I can squat clean, which is only about 80% of my BW. The issue here is clearly getting under the bar, and to be honest there is a lot of fear involved when dropping under substantial weight, even though I know I'm strong enough to handle it. So I've been doing a lot of hang cleans with about 55%-60% BW and I can receive the bar fairly solidly in the hole, which is a huge confidence builder.

Today I was power cleaning and feeling really good, so I decided to test my max. I did triples up to 60% BW, then singles in increments of 10lbs. I just found that as the bar started approaching my body weight, the whole feel of the lift changed and not just the perception of heaviness. I tried to keep my mechanics the same, and was I achieving more than sufficient bar height to get under the bar in a power position, but I had a lot of misses. I finally topped out at 98% BW, which I caught somewhat sloppily just under parallel and which buried me, but I did manage to stand up with it. What struck me on this final lift was that all the technique work in the world didn't prepare me for the "feel" of taking a bar close to my own weight through the second pull and catching it in the hole. I can only imagine that as the bar gets heavier than the lifter the leverage shifts which might be causing this different feel. Is this a real consideration or do I just have to get used to lifting heavier?

Greg Says: I suspect that what's happening is that your balance during the lift is forward at all weights and you simply aren't aware of it when the weights are light because they're not heavy enough to influence your position and balance further. That is, with 50% of your bodyweight, you can do just about anything and get away with it—an errant bar is easy to pull back to you later in the lift because your own bodyweight is enough to remain the anchor in the system. As the bar approaches your own weight, it has just as much control over you as you do over it. In this case, the errant bar pulls you out of position and you're unable to simply muscle it back into place as needed later.

Another possibility (which could be occurring together with the previous) is that your mechanics are in fact changing as the weight increases. Most likely, this would be your hips moving up faster than your shoulders as you lift the bar from the floor. As a powerlifter, it's very likely that you're posterior-chain dominant, which means that it will be hard for you to open your knee joint from a small angle because your quads are relatively weak. The body will shift the work to whatever is strongest, and in such a case, it does this by opening the knee without opening the hip to create a larger knee angle without moving the weight very much. This then puts the knee at a larger angle that the quads can continue opening under the full load and transfers more of the weight to the strong hip extensors. This can have two effects that will cause you a lot of trouble and certainly change the feel of the lift: shift your weight forward farther over your feet, and increase the moment arm on the hip. The first makes it impossible to finish your pull properly and forces you to chase the bar forward rather than being able to move it up and yourself down. The second makes the extension of the hips more difficult and consequently slower, making it tougher to get the quick explosion at the top of the pull that you need to have a chance to get under the bar.

Perform snatch and clean deadlifts and halting deadlifts with no more weight than what allows you to keep the proper upright posture. Focus on pushing with the legs to move the bar up to the thighs and shifting back toward your heels and staying there all the way to the top. This will not only train you in terms of skill to pull correctly, but will begin to strengthen you in the proper posture. Remember that as the weight increases, your body will always revert to the positions in which it's strongest. You can also combine halting deadlifts with snatches and cleans in a number of ways. The simplest is to perform 1-3 halting deadlifts followed by a snatch or clean. Another is to perform the halting deadlift and rather than returning to the floor, performing the snatch or clean straight from the paused position. This can work really well, but I will usually have a lifter follow a rep like this with a normal rep from the floor to help prevent them from developing a habit of pausing during a lift or hitching.

Finally, more front squats for the clean and overhead squats for the snatch will strengthen the positions and boost your confidence.

Claudia Asks: Dear Greg, Aimee or both: I was doing CrossFit for two years but got tired of being constantly injured. My CrossFit gym started a specialized two day a week Olympic lifting class. I have been in the class since March and love it. Even though I'm 37 years old and never lifted weights, I've gained strength and technique. My husband and I are planning to have a baby soon and I was wondering what type of workout should I do while pregnant that would allow me to stay fit and strong and come back to class within a reasonable time after giving birth. I haven't seen any pregnant woman doing Olympic lifting, so I'm assuming it's probably not very safe? Or would it be possible to stay in class for the first few months and just lighten loads etc? Thanks.

Greg Says: Training during pregnancy is a really individual thing. The most important rule is to never do anything you're not comfortable with. Unless you have some pregnancy-related medical complication with specific contraindications, you should be fine with most movements that don't involve bouncing or ballistic loading, the former for obvious reasons, and the latter because your connective tissue will begin loosening as your pregnancy continues, making your joints more lax and susceptible to injury (this means no kipping pull-ups!). Obvious things like not lying on your back or stomach are out too. Generally women train pretty normally during the first trimester, then begin back off significantly during the second, and the third is pretty low-level work.

In terms of lifting, doing controlled movements like overhead squats, back squats, front squats, deadlifts and pressing variations should be fine as long as you stick with light weights and don't over-pressurize your trunk (just keep breathing normally as much as possible). After the first trimester, I wouldn't snatch, clean or jerk.

We have a collection in the store of three articles from three different women who detail their experiences training while pregnant. Each took a somewhat different approach, but each continued to be active and was very successful. In any case, stay in touch with your doctor and make sure you discuss what you're doing or plan to do.

Andy Asks: I have just purchased and am reading through your book now. Its is a great teaching tool. Thanks for it! I was curious about the hook grip you teach. I think i understand the technique, however it not really working out. The strength of the grip for me is very weak. I have been using it a month and just have trouble keeping that grip. Do I just need to give it more time? I have pretty stubby fingers. Is it just not optimal for everyone? I'm like 5'9- 5'10 (depends on who's asking). 83kg.

Just thought I'd try and ask an expert. I understand it's value in that it can provide for more gains in multiple lifts. So i would like to get it down. Would it be more practical to do this in a volume phase of work to be able to work with decreased weight? Thanks again.

Greg Says: The hook grip can be tricky initially, especially for individuals with smaller hands, and even more so for those smaller handed individuals whose hands are also thick. The short answer is: Make it work. There's a reason that every weightlifter in the world uses the hook grip, and that's simply that when you're accelerating a barbell as you do in the snatch and clean, you cannot maintain your grip without it.

When you start feeling sorry for yourself, just remember that there are 56 kg (124 lb) men who snatch and clean with the hook grip on the same 28 mm barbell that the rest of us use. Halil Mutlu snatched 138 kg at 56 kg. If someone with hands that small can hold onto a weight that big with a snatch grip, you can find a way to manage.

First, when you're first setting your grip, push the webbing between your thumb and index finger into the bar as deep as possible, and then wrap the thumb and fingers. This should help you get a bit more reach with the thumb.

For most people, there is some stretching that needs to occur before the hook grip feels really secure. The best way to accomplish this is to simply use the hook grip every time you're pulling a bar. Your thumbs will stretch out a bit and your hands will become conditioned to the position, and it will eventually start feeling much more comfortable.

You can also stretch directly with what I call the girl punch stretch (no offense intended - none of my female lifters would ever punch someone this way). Make a fist with your thumb tucked tightly inside and ulnar deviate your hand; that is, tilt your hand away from the thumb side. You should feel a stretch around the base of your thumb and probably a little up into your wrist as well. You can also flex the wrist from this position to get an additional and somewhat different stretch.

If you really want to torture yourself, you can do heavy deadlifts with a hook grip. This will stretch your out and strengthen the grip with less chance of a sudden slip than you would have in a snatch or clean, but it will also be painful (most people feel like their thumbnails are being crushed in a vice).

Finally, you can try taping your thumbs. Make sure you use elastic tape so your joints can move freely. Sometimes tape will have a bit more friction against the bar and make your grip feel more secure.

In any case, keep using it as much as possible and as frequently as possible and it will improve.

Maguid Asks: Hi Greg et al., I am up in Toronto, running a Crossfit and working towards the goals of increasing my capacity and technical proficiency across all of the modalities under the CF umbrella.

I have been on the 2-phase cycle you programmed in April 2009, with some modifications on the volume of course. Five weeks in, I have seen some huge gains across the board! I am planning for the next phase of my training a little early knowing how fast the remaining weeks will fly by, and I have a couple of quick questions:

1. Looking at the current 18 week program, I'm wondering what the rationale is behind it. I'm noticing a lot of RMs each day similar to the strength by feel program. How does this one differ from strength by feel exactly?

2. On the training side, since starting the 2-phase cycle I have developed occasional irritation/swelling in one of my knees, presumably from some positioning issues I have with the squat. I got knee sleeves and those help, as well as working to really make space for the joint with mobility work before training sessions. It has improved, but I'm hoping you might have some tips or experience with managing knee issues.

I love the site, and read the articles regularly. I especially loved Jocelyn's kicking the metcon habit article. I found it to be mature and thoughtful, as well as honest. Thanks a lot!

THE PORTABLE GREG EVERETT

Greg Says: The 3-phase 18-week cycle is similar to the strength by feel cycle in the sense that I don't prescribe weights as often and instead just prescribe reps and sets with the expectation that the lifter will find the appropriate weight each day. I honestly prefer prescribing weights, but the reality with programming for a bunch of athletes I don't know and never see is that I can't do that with any accuracy. With my own lifters, it's possible, and even then, I don't always prescribe weights; sometimes I will prescribe a range of percentages and always explain what I expect them to do.

The 18-week cycle is broken into 3 distinct phases that each has a different emphasis. The first phase is focused on building squatting and pressing strength (the latter might be better called overhead strength, as this includes jerk and snatch-related work); the second focuses more on pulling strength; and the last focuses on the classic lifts. The first two phases taper and test maxes on the last week, both as a way to keep an eye on progress, to give a break from the volume, and to make sure we're not going too long without feeling heavy snatches and clean & jerks. The strength by feel cycle is like a more generalized version of the above. That is, there aren't distinct emphases at any given point. And of course it's half the duration. This cycle is more appropriate for more beginning lifters. I tend to post programs with fairly high volume, which will often be more than many who follow the site can manage, but I have expectations that they will modify it as necessary (as you state you did with the 2-phase cycle).

Regarding the knee, I genuinely believe that the only reason a knee ever hurts from weightlifting is if something is being done incorrectly. There is nothing inherently damaging about the movements themselves. That being said, people who do every lift perfectly and have no strength or flexibility imbalances don't exist, so there will always be potential for the aggravation of joints.

Since your description of the problem is vague (and I'm not a medical professional), I can only make guesses regarding what the problem is. Typically, as you said, there is an issue with the squat movement being improper in the sense that the knee is not able to move smoothly through the range of motion with a perfect balance of forces on it. This could be something as simple as a tight ITB that tugs the kneecap to the outside a bit too much and as a result causes some abnormal friction in the joint, which could cause enough irritation for some minor swelling. Or you might have some scar tissue built up somewhere in the joint capsule that creates a similar problem. In any case, the smart course of action is to try to identify the cause by tracking when the swelling occurs—e.g. after what movements, what time of day, what activity you do before and after that may affect it, how much or how you warm-up, etc.

In addition, I like doing a shotgun approach to cover as many bases as possible. If something in there works, you will eventually figure out what it was, and any superfluous work isn't likely to harm you. Tons of foam rolling on all aspects of the quads, hamstrings and adductors; extra work with a lacrosse ball or similar on the ITB; stretch the quads and hip flexors aggressively pre- and post-workout.

Post workout, stretch all the hip musculature as well—we want to make sure you're not crooked. Doing unilateral stretches should make it pretty obvious if something is tighter on one side than the other.

And finally, try to identify any movement dysfunction during squatting or movements involving squatting, e.g. that knee shifting inward or outward, always throwing that foot farther out than the other during a clean or snatch, or that foot being rotated out more or less than the other, etc., and work to correct this through stretching, strengthening and technical work.

Christine Asks: I just had a private session with my coach at Crossfit Inland Empire and my major problem with cleans is that the bar hits the top of my shoulders after I get my elbow out in front.

Are there any suggestions to fix this? My coach says that I still round the bar out in front of me instead of keeping it close to my body. How high is it suggested to pull the bar up for the clean?

Thanks for your time and any input you're able to provide. :)

Greg Says: Very common problem and a big limiter for the clean. Basically, if the bar is crashing down onto your shoulders, you're losing your connection to it somehow at some point. Figuring out when and why will allow you to correct the problem.

If your coach is correct in saying that the bar swings forward during the turnover, there are a couple possible causes, and most likely, it's a combination of more than one. First, the movement of your arms and the body during the pull under itself are incorrect. Most likely, this means allowing your elbows to move backward and to stay in toward your sides. Instead, you need to turn the elbows out as far as you can right from the start of the lift and keep them oriented that way until you're done pulling yourself down toward the bar and it's time to bring the elbows around the bar and up into the rack position. I will emphasize this point because so often people dismiss its importance. Rotate the elbows to the sides. All the way. Not a little bit. Until they don't rotate any more. This doesn't mean round your shoulders forward, by the way. Internally rotate the arm with neutral (protraction/retraction) and somewhat depressed shoulder blades.

The second most likely cause is that you're not staying over the bar long enough and as a consequence, it's hitting low on your thighs and getting pushed forward as you finish your extension, which you likely can't finish well because of this. Aim to keep the shoulders slightly in front of the bar until it's at the upper thigh and only then initiate the final explosion of the knees and hips. This will allow the knees to shift forward as they should naturally and the bar to move back into you rather than hanging up on the legs as they're moving forward. If you do this well, the mechanics of the pull under actually matter less (but don't neglect them).

THE PORTABLE GREG EVERETT

You can practice muscle cleans with very light weights to get the feel for this. When I say light, I mean light enough that the turnover can be done quickly and with little resistance. Focus on making the bar move straight up your torso and smoothly onto your shoulders—you'll quickly find that the only way this is possible is by pulling the elbows high and to the sides.

I wrote an article of somewhat ridiculous length about this very topic that you can read on the website called Improving the Clean through a Better Turnover. That should help you further diagnose the cause and determine the best way to resolve the problem.

Bruce Asks: So I am in the middle of a life changing/saving journey, I have dropped 100 pounds in the past year through nutrition and Crossfit. During this journey I have found a love of the barbell and moving heavy weight. My question is this: At 36 am I too old to see significant gains in my lifts? I recently transitioned from a pure CrossFit cycle to a mixed strength/CrossFit cycle, I have an Oly lifting coach who is working with me on my form and technique, and I have the drive to compete. What I don't want to do is set goals that are not obtainable. So at 36, should I just focus on general fitness, or is it possible to still see significant weight gains in my lifts. Thank You!

Greg Says: You will be able to realize considerable gains if you learn the lifts and train appropriately. At 36, you won't recover as quickly from training and won't be able to handle as much volume as your early-20s counterparts, but that doesn't mean you're hopeless. I coach masters lifters from 40 to 55 years old, all of whom still make progress even on strength lifts, not just Olympic lifts through technical improvements, don't get injured, compete and enjoy training.

To set goals, I would suggest looking at the masters records for your age & weight category get an idea of what's possible and work from that. Keep in mind that in your age category, there are some very good lifters who have maintained pretty well from their senior lifter careers, so don't set goals based on the numbers of such outliers. Take into consideration all the obligations of life that will limit your training time and recovery time, e.g. work and family, and also your late start with weightlifting. And of course, the more you want to make gains in weightlifting, the less CrossFit you need to do, so make sure your training choices reflect your goals and priorities.

Make mobility and injury prevention an emphasis—nothing will slow you down like injuries and flexibility limitations.

KJ Asks: I found your website about 6 weeks ago, but bought your Oly book awhile back - it's fantastic! Last March, I discovered Olympic Lifting through my CrossFit gym here in Iowa, and was making some pretty good gains until I blew out my left ACL on August 8th. Had surgery Sept. 13, and am now 12 weeks post surgery, and cleared to do many things - low box jumps, deadlifts, squats, and the like. The one thing I won't be cleared to do for awhile is full O-lifts - my surgeon doesn't want me to be shifting my feet from the starting position to the receiving position (with weight) for another 8 weeks, at least. I'm trying to get around this by doing partial movements - high pulls, heaving snatch balance, push presses, and the like, but was wondering if you had any advice in terms of programming (good substitutions for the full/power lifts), and what (if any) your experience has been with athletes post-ACL surgery. Strength is my goal here. Thanks in advance! Keep rockin' over there at Catalyst! Love your stuff!

Greg Says: First and foremost, always get your doc's approval before you add anything to training. There aren't many things as frustrating as getting set back on recovery time through aggravation of an incompletely healed injury or surgery.

Next, my question would be how you blew out your knee, because that may give you some good guidance on what you need to work on as you come back. Based on your email, I'm not sure if you injured the knee actually lifting or doing CrossFit (or, also pretty likely, blew it out during lifting after having set it up for the injury through CF abuse). But if it was entirely the result of lifting, there is a problem with something you're doing: lifting itself shouldn't be placing that kind of stress on your ACL. I would go back and evaluate your squat mechanics, especially during cleans and snatches, and look for moments at which your knee is not hinging squarely, but experiencing some kind of rotation or lateral stress. Big thing I would look for is having a squat stance that is both too wide and with the toes too straight forward.

In any case, as you come back, prioritize the re-establishment of proper mechanics through a lot of deliberate positional work. I would squat daily, not with a lot of weight, but using the frequency and volume to build up connective tissue strength and ingrain the perfect motor pattern. Consider using pause squats some of the time not only to allow more strength development in the deepest position, but also to further reinforce proper mechanics in the recovery.

Spend plenty of time preparing to train with foam rolling, necessary stretching and generally getting warm and moving fluidly. Use standard knee strengthening protocols that focus on VMO strength and hip strength/stability: exercises like terminal knee extensions with a band, backward sled pulling, Peterson step-ups, and 1 and ¼ squats for the VMO; mini-band squats, X-band walks and clamshells for hip stability; and things like unilateral bent-knee balancing on an air pad for general stability and proprioception work.

If strength is your goal, focus on strength work. Squats, pull and deadlift variations, press variations, heaving snatch balance, and muscle snatches and cleans. You might also try doing the lifts without moving your feet. Start with the feet in your receiving position, keep the weights light, and force yourself to maintain contact with the floor and receive the bar tightly and with total control of the squat mechanics. This will just allow you to keep a feel for the lifts until you're cleared to do them.

Matt Asks: I bought the Olympic weightlifting book by Tommy Kono and watched a few of his videos. I noticed that he recommends to have your shoulders pushed forwards, lats spread when doing snatches and cleans. I trained that way for a while until my shoulder started to bother me. My chiropractor said that it was bad for my shoulders to lift that way and that they should be pulled back and down. I also noticed that some Olympic trainers recommend to have your shoulders pulled back to ensure a good arch. So I'm a bit confused as to what is the best way.

Greg Says: First of all, I have a huge amount of respect for Kono and in no way should anything I say be interpreted to suggest otherwise. In the start and pull of the snatch and clean, I teach lifters to keep the shoulders approximately neutral with regard to retraction/protraction. We definitely don't want to try to retract, partly because it will typically be impossible to reach the bar with a good body position, but also because it's unlikely the athlete would be able to maintain that scapular position under the load anyway. However, I don't believe there is a need to actively or intentionally protract either. Depending on how a lifter is built, their flexibility, and the particulars of their starting position, some protraction may occur unavoidably, and this is fine.

The lifter needs to be concerned more with arching the back. Part of this effort should involve forcefully engaging the lats. This will not only help extend the upper back, but will also pull the bar inward toward the lifter so it can be controlled. This effort to engage the lats will depress the shoulder blades somewhat, and will retract them at least somewhat from the position they would be in without such lat activation. This is the position we want to achieve and maintain during the pull.

Ed Asks: I've been training Bulgarian style. I say style because I've only incorporated an aspect of their training methodology. The program is merely squatting. I've backed off of Oly Lifting since I feel I need to get some coaching before I continue. So I squat to max every single day, only once a day. After the initial 2 months where I say my daily maxes drop significantly, I am now in the 181+kilo club (of course high bar ATG style). My question is how do you supplement or should I? I have access to a GHD and a few rudimentary training tools. For now my goals are to get strong as F*@% with the caveat not to get fat as F*@%. I'm not shredding just don't want to flirt with metabolic derangement. Can I throw in some metcon style stuff in 5-10 min. windows? Do I need to balance stuff out with specific mobility drills? I fear that given the daily toll that squatting takes, especially on the soft tissue, that I may be primed for a tear if I dip into metcons? I don't know so I'm simply spit-balling.

Greg Says: I don't think there's any need to do metCons in order to not get fat; if you're getting fat, your nutrition is out of order. Generally my standpoint is that you train for physical abilities; you eat for weight and body composition. Granted, there is some crossover, but if you have certain performance goals, keep your training oriented that way as much as possible.

If all you're doing is squatting, then yes, do more. But it doesn't have to be conditioning work. You can do basic bodybuilding and strength work that will help your goal of getting stronger rather than interfere with it. There is a large variety of upper body pushing and pulling exercises that can be done with a barbell. If you have limited time, you can superset exercises, and this will also give you a bit of a conditioning response—just don't push it to CrossFit style efforts. I would especially avoid leg-centric conditioning work if your goal is squat strength and you're already squatting heavy daily. Stick to upper body and ab/back exercises and if you do any additional leg work, make it relatively light unilateral exercises like lunge or split squat variations.

Chad Asks: First, thanks for all that you do for all of us who have found Catalyst Athletics, the Paleo Solution Podcast with RW, and more.

A bit of background. I'm a 40 year old male who has been involved in athletics for my entire life. I played competitive high school ice hockey, got into various outdoor pursuits in collage, and for the past 15 plus years have "trained" in various modalities…some lifting (everything from Bigger, Faster, Stronger to Body for Life to…more recently…intense circuit training/ boot camp), cycling, recreational ice hockey, mountain biking, a bit of running, you get the picture.

Starting in August of 2010, I joined Cape CrossFit, a box in Cape Town, South Africa. We lived there until June 2011, and I loved the experience at CCF. I competed in the open, and finished, but ended up hurting my back on the clean squat and jerk workout. Consequently, I backed off training in the spring.

Upon my return to the states, my wife and I put together our own Cross Fit style home gym (at our house in Idaho where we spend our summers). Wanting to work on my mobility (lots of desk time = really tight hips in particular), I starting the novice programming for Starting Strength. I followed this until we returned east to our new "permanent" home in New Hampshire, where we live and work at a boarding school. Once we had finished the move, I re-started the Starting Strength novice programming. I am currently seven session. he lifts are still relatively easy and my form is solid, if not perfect. My latest numbers are: Squat - 205lbs, 3X5; Press - 110lbs, 3X5; Power Clean - 135lbs, 5X3; Bench - 160 lbs, 3X5, and Deadlift - 275, 1X5. On non-starting strength days, I usually do some combination of mobility, dynamic warmup, and high intensity (short) intervals on the erg or bike.

In terms of nutrition, I recently completed a clean paleo month, which helped to lean out significantly. I haven't measured body fat, but I suspect I'm around 10-12%. I weigh 170-175 and am 6 ft. even, with a fairly l lanky build (fat appears on the love handles first).

My goals are to get stronger and then to become proficient in the realm of Olympic Lifting. Continued mobility improvement and general health and well being are also important.

I'm considering starting up with one of the Catalyst programs. Can you recommend a program to begin with? My build is such (long in the limbs) that I will never be an awesome or even competitive oly lifter, but I still believe that work in this realm will have high pay offs for me in reaching my goals.

Any advice you can provide would be much appreciated!

THE PORTABLE GREG EVERETT

Greg Says: Because it sounds like you still have room to grow with the SS program, I would suggest continuing that until you really tap it out. No reason to move on before you've completely exhausted it. However, this would be a good time to start working on mobility and skill for the Olympic lifts so that when it's time to move to a new program, you'll be able to do it properly.

On the non-SS days, continue with the mobility work and intervals, but add some Olympic-lift-related barbell work such as overhead squats, snatch balance variations, split jerk position work, front squats, snatch and clean segment deadlifts, and muscle snatches and cleans. This should all be light and easy (probably all with an empty barbell) to allow you to do as much volume as you want and feel is needed without taxing you to any significant degree. This is all movement practice and mobility work.

When you're done with SS, I would suggest using the Classic/Position Cycle on the website. This cycle uses a lot of technical work to help you develop and reinforce proper movement. It's a lot of work, but it's relatively light, and it can be made as light as needed to allow you to manage the volume. The squats and assistance strength work will keep your strength up even if you keep the majority of the training pretty light. There are videos of all of the exercises on the site.

After that cycle, you should be well prepared to take on just about any other on the site.

Francois Asks: Hi Greg, First of all pardon any errors in my English, I'm French. I've discovered oly lifting thanks to your book, and started practicing on my own since there is no club close enough to where I work. So my technique probably was quite awful, but I used videos to have online critique of my form whenever possible. And most of all, I really enjoyed the sport. I was not doing a pure oly routine, rather a mix of oly and powerlifting.

Last year I've been diagnosed with a herniated disk, L5-S1. The only advice I got from physicians was to stop weightlifting, squats, press, deadlift, etc. I've since then switched to weighted chins, weighed dips, bench... But I really miss the clean and jerk. And one year later, although the pain has mostly subdued, I still have occurrences of flaring lower back. I've tried split squats, but even that seemed to trigger pain past 60-70kg (although it might be unrelated). Same with front squats past 80-90kg.

In retrospect, I believe what caused my hernia, on top of a probable genetic weakness, was tail tuck at the bottom of the squat. It's something I couldn't improve whatever hip mobility stretches I did, so I always had a bit of tail tuck. Now if I attempt to squat in any way, I simply don't go as deep.

I've read all of Stuart McGill books, and am currently doing mainly calisthenics and planks to gain spine stability. I also contemplate doing weighted planks to further improve spine stability under load, as well as overhead squats (something I've never done).

I'm not asking for medical advice, rather for past experience about this kind of problems, which I wager is quite common. Is there any hope, or should I accept that oly lifting is forever out of reach for me? And what kind of exercises or stretches can I do to improve my situation?

Thanks for your time, and hopefully, any answer on your part.

Greg Says: This is definitely a tough one, as what works for one person with this injury will not work for another. In any case, I would very strongly suggest you find a medical practitioner (such as a chiropractor who also does soft tissue work) who has experience working with athletes and understands the mechanics of strength training. Having a good relationship with someone like this is invaluable when trying to come back from such an injury. Regular work with this practitioner can keep everything in check as well as help you gauge whether or not certain practices in your training are helping or hurting. So, first and foremost, work with a medical professional, be smart and be safe.

Making trunk stability and strength the primary focus is a good idea. Make sure you're approaching all aspects of trunk stability, however, not just the abdominals; strengthen the back and improve mobility in the hips and thoracic spine. The lower back commonly becomes the point that makes up for immobility in surrounding areas. If the hips are not mobile enough, the needed movement will come from the lumbar spine; even limited mobility in the thoracic spine and shoulder girdle can force hypermobility in the lower back. You apparently have tight hips and are aware of your inability to maintain lumbar extension in the bottom of a squat; I agree with you that this is a very likely cause of the problem.

So, the first priority is strengthening the trunk's ability to maintain a neutral spine position under load. Planks, side planks and supine planks (for the back) are a good foundation. You can add weight IF you're able to hold a perfect position for a considerable period of time; if you can't hold a perfect plank for over a minute without struggling, don't bother adding weight. I would also add some unweighted back extensions with a limited range of motion, isometric hold at the top, and a focus on maintaining tight abs. Try to set up a 45-degree back extension or glute-ham developer such that the fulcrum pad is actually under your abs instead of your hips. Let the spine flex slightly without allowing the lumbar spine to get past about flat (i.e. no actual flexion there), then extend slowly until you're just beyond neutral (no extreme hyperextension in the lower back). Keep the abs tight throughout the movement to help prevent hyperextension. Hold the extended position for 5-10 seconds before lowering for the next rep. You will probably not be able to do many reps initially with this hold, and you may not be able to hold that long. Start with what you can do and build up gradually. If you feel any pain, stop immediately.

The next priority is improving flexibility so you're able to move through a better range of motion at the hips and ankles, which will allow you to squat to better depth while maintaining proper spine position. When it comes to stretching, in my opinion, the only "trick" is consistency and frequency; that is, stretch as much as you can as often as you can and do it every single day. Stretch the hips in all directions; don't just focus on the hamstrings and adductors as many do.

Once you've developed the trunk strength and hip mobility to sit into squat with a perfect spine position, I would reintroduce back squats very conservatively. On each rep, focus on pressurizing the trunk and locking it into position tightly. Start with an empty bar and do only as many reps as you can with no loss of position—initially, that might be only 2-3. Do a few sets along with your other training. Over time, build up until you can do 3-4 sets of 10 reps with perfect positioning. Once you reach that point, assuming you still have no pain (which you should if you're still doing this), start adding weight incrementally to one squat session per week. The other days of the week, stick with unweighted or empty barbell squats only as both a way to maintain mobility and to practice the movement. At this point, you can reintroduce the deadlift in the same manner—never compromise perfect spinal position. When you've spend a good deal of time rebuilding your foundation with the squat and deadlift, are strong in the proper positions, and are pain-free consistently, you can start reintroducing the Olympic lifts, although I would be extremely conservative with weight and volume, and starting with power and even hang-power variations is probably wise.

This process may take a long time, but stick with it. Better to invest a lot of time and effort into rehabbing yourself than throwing in the towel and never doing what you like to do again. Good luck.

Justin Asks: Hey Greg... Wondering if you could give me some thoughts on combining Olympic Programming while still making WOD progress... I realize getting back to the strength I had while just being a competitive weightlifter only is probably not an option, but was curious what your thoughts were on trying to work things in along with metcon programming, etc... Two or maybe in this case three heads are better than one... :) Here is what I was thinking of as of now...

2 Days On / 1 Day Off x 3 Cycles Before Repeating With WOD Constantly Changing From Cycle To Cycle

1st Cycle:

Day One:
1. Snatch (Rep Max Work 2-5 Reps)(Keep Same Rep Scheme For Three Weeks, Building Up Work Set Percentages EA Wk...Ex... 90% 3RM, 95% 3RM, Last Week - Retest 3RM
2. Deadlift
3. Assistance Work
4. Metcon

Day Two:
1. Skill Work (Rings, Etc)
2. Weighted OH Movement (1-5 Reps)
3. Metcon

2nd Cycle:

Day One:
1. Clean & Jerk Variation (Power, Full, Jerk, No Jerk, Etc)
2. Front Squat (5/3/1 Program)
3. PC/Heavy Rowing
4. Metcon (Maybe)

Day Two:
1. Olympic Work (Lighter Weight, From Blocks, 3 Position, Etc)
2. Metcon

3rd Cycle:

Day One:
1. Snatch - Singles Up to 90, 95 OR Heavy Single
2. Clean & Jerk - Same
3. Back Squat (Russian Squat Program)
4. Gymnastics Work

Day Two:
1. Maybe 2 Workout Day... Mostly Conditioning Based Day With A Weakness Included

Just A Rough Idea of My thoughts... Any comments? Suggestions? Thanks in advance!

Greg Says: First, I would say that generally the plan looks pretty good. You're addressing just about everything you presumably need to work on. You have a heavier, higher-volume day followed by a lighter, lower-volume day, which is a good setup. You don't specify the details of the metCons listed, so I don't know how that will work. This is a pretty good amount of work, even with a rest day every third day, so if those conditioning workouts are long and brutal, you may find it's too much. What I would suggest is keeping them fairly brief in the first two cycles, then doing a short one first on day two of the third cycle, and a long, tough one second on day two of the third cycle; make that your only really nasty conditioning workout in that nine-day period.

The other thing that stands out is the squats: you have one day of front squats based on the 5/3/1 program and one day of back squats based on the Russian squat program. First, you're mixing two programs, which is always tricky and usually not effective. In this case, you're mixing a program that runs on a 4-week cycle with one that runs on a 6-week cycle into a program that runs on a 9-day cycle; 5/3/1 has you squat once weekly and the RSP has you squat three times weekly. I'm not saying it's not possible, but it's unclear how you plan to make that work. I would say that it's overcomplicating things. I would front squat one day and back squat one day, and select the weight and volume like you are for your Olympic lifts. For example, back squat heavy and with high volume, and front squat with somewhat lower volume and intensity; build for 3 cycles and retest. That may not be the ultimate strength program, but keep in mind this isn't weightlifting anymore—you're doing a mix of a lot of different things and simple tends to work just fine in that case, and you won't be working at your maximum strength capacity.

16480880R00105

Printed in Great Britain
by Amazon